T0348599

Hematologic and Oncologic Emergencies

Editors

COLIN G. KAIDE
SARAH B. DUBBS

EMERGENCY MEDICINE CLINICS OF NORTH AMERICA

www.emed.theclinics.com

Consulting Editor
AMAL MATTU

August 2018 • Volume 36 • Number 3

ELSEVIER

1600 John F. Kennedy Boulevard • Suite 1800 • Philadelphia, Pennsylvania, 19103-2899

http://www.theclinics.com

EMERGENCY MEDICINE CLINICS OF NORTH AMERICA Volume 36, Number 3
August 2018 ISSN 0733-8627, ISBN-13: 978-0-323-61384-2

Editor: Colleen Dietzler
Developmental Editor: Casey Potter

Emergency Medicine Clinics of North America (ISSN 0733-8627) is published quarterly by Elsevier Inc., 360 Park Avenue South, New York, NY, 10010-1710. Months of issue are February, May, August, and November. Business and Editorial Offices: 1600 John F. Kennedy Boulevard, Suite 1800, Philadelphia, PA 19103-2899. Customer Service Office: 6277 Sea Harbor Drive, Orlando, FL 32887-4800. Periodicals postage paid at New York, NY, and additional mailing offices. Subscription prices are $100.00 per year (US students), $336.00 per year (US individuals), $644.00 per year (US institutions), $220.00 per year (international students), $455.00 per year (international individuals), $791.00 per year (international institutions), $220.00 per year (Canadian students), $405.00 per year (Canadian individuals), and $791.00 per year (Canadian institutions). International air speed delivery is included in all *Clinics'* subscription prices. All prices are subject to change without notice. **POSTMASTER:** Send address changes to *Emergency Medicine Clinics of North America*, Elsevier Periodicals Customer Service, 11830 Westline Industrial Drive, St. Louis, MO 63146. Customer Service (orders, claims, online, change of address): Elsevier Periodicals **Customer Service, 11830 Westline Industrial Drive, St. Louis, MO 63146. Tel: 1-800-654-2452 (U.S. and Canada); 314-453-7041 (outside U.S. and Canada). Fax: 314-453-5170. E-mail: journalscustomerservice-usa@elsevier.com (for print support)**; journalsonlinesupport-usa@elsevier.com **(for online support).**

Reprints. For copies of 100 or more of articles in this publication, please contact the Commercial Reprints Department, Elsevier Inc., 360 Park Avenue South, New York, NY 10010-1710. Tel.: 212-633-3874; Fax: 212-633-3820; E-mail: reprints@elsevier.com.

Emergency Medicine Clinics of North America is covered in *MEDLINE/PubMed (Index Medicus), Current Contents/Clinical Medicine, EMBASE/Excerpta Medica, BIOSIS, SciSearch, CINAHL, ISI/BIOMED,* and *Research Alert.*

Printed in the United States of America.

Contributors

CONSULTING EDITOR

AMAL MATTU, MD
Professor and Vice Chair of Education, Department of Emergency Medicine, University of Maryland School of Medicine, Baltimore, Maryland

EDITORS

COLIN G. KAIDE, MD, FACEP, FAAEM
Associate Professor of Emergency Medicine, Specialist in Hyperbaric Medicine, Core Faculty, Emergency Medicine Residency, Department of Emergency Medicine, Wexner Medical Center, The Ohio State University, Columbus, Ohio

SARAH B. DUBBS, MD, FAAEM
Assistant Residency Program Director, Clinical Assistant Professor, Department of Emergency Medicine, University of Maryland School of Medicine, Baltimore, Maryland

AUTHORS

ANGELA IRENE CARRICK, DO, FACOEP
Associate Program Director, Norman Regional Emergency Medicine Residency, Board Certified Emergency Medicine Physician, Norman Regional Hospital, Norman, Oklahoma

STEPHANIE CHARSHAFIAN, MD
Division of Emergency Medicine, Washington University School of Medicine, Barnes-Jewish Hospital, St Louis, Missouri

HOLLY BRIANN COSTNER, DO
Core Faculty, Norman Regional Emergency Medicine Residency, Board Certified Emergency Medicine Physician, Norman Regional Hospital, Norman, Oklahoma

MATTHEW DAVIS, DO
Core Clinical Faculty, Emergency Medicine Residency, Norman Regional Health Systems, Norman, Oklahoma

LUCA R. DELATORE, MD
Assistant Professor, Department of Emergency Medicine, Medical Director, Emergency Services, Emergency Oncology Fellowship Director, Wexner Medical Center at The Ohio State University, Columbus, Ohio

SARAH B. DUBBS, MD, FAAEM
Assistant Residency Program Director, Clinical Assistant Professor, Department of Emergency Medicine, University of Maryland School of Medicine, Baltimore, Maryland

IMAD EL MAJZOUB, MD
Fellow, Department of Emergency Medicine, The University of Texas MD Anderson Cancer Center, Houston, Texas

GEREMIHA EMERSON, MD
Assistant Professor, Department of Emergency Medicine, Wexner Medical Center, The Ohio State University, Columbus, Ohio

AKILESH P. HONASOGE, MD
Departments of Emergency Medicine and Internal Medicine, University of Maryland Medical Center, Baltimore, Maryland

COLIN G. KAIDE, MD, FACEP, FAAEM
Associate Professor of Emergency Medicine, Specialist in Hyperbaric Medicine, Core Faculty, Emergency Medicine Residency, Department of Emergency Medicine, Wexner Medical Center, The Ohio State University, Columbus, Ohio

ALEX KOYFMAN, MD
Department of Emergency Medicine, The University of Texas Southwestern Medical Center, Dallas, Texas

STEPHEN Y. LIANG, MD, MPHS
Divisions of Emergency Medicine and Infectious Diseases, Washington University School of Medicine, St Louis, Missouri

BRIT LONG, MD
Department of Emergency Medicine, San Antonio Military Medical Center, Fort Sam Houston, Texas

LINDSEY PICARD, MD
Resident Physician, Department of Emergency Medicine, University of Rochester, Rochester, New York

MICHAEL PORTER, MD
Core Faculty, Department of Emergency Medicine, Norman Regional Hospital, Norman, Oklahoma

MICHAEL G. PURCELL, MD
Fellow, Department of Emergency Medicine, Wexner Medical Center, The Ohio State University, Columbus, Ohio

DANIEL J. SESSIONS, MD
Attending Physician, Emergency Medicine, San Antonio Uniformed Services Health Education Consortium, Fort Sam Houston, Texas

ERICA M. SIMON, DO, MHA
Attending Physician, Emergency Medicine, San Antonio Uniformed Services Health Education Consortium, Fort Sam Houston, Texas

KATHLEEN STEPHANOS, MD
Clinical Instructor of Emergency Medicine, Departments of Pediatrics and Emergency Medicine, University of Rochester, Rochester, New York

MATTHEW J. STREITZ, MD
Attending Physician, Emergency Medicine, San Antonio Uniformed Services Health Education Consortium, Fort Sam Houston, Texas

SHELLY ZIMMERMAN, DO, FACOEP
Director of Medical Education, Medical Student Clerkship Director, Core Clinical Faculty, Emergency Medicine Residency, Norman Regional Health Systems, Norman, Oklahoma; Adjunct Clinical Faculty, Oklahoma State University College of Osteopathic Medicine, Tulsa, Oklahoma

Contents

> The latest cancer agents, collectively known as cancer immunotherapy, have tremendously increased the armamentarium against cancer. Their targeted mechanisms seem ideal, but they do come with complications. As these therapies become more widespread, emergency physicians everywhere must be aware of the immune-related adverse events that can occur and be ready to identify and coordinate treatment. This article provides the emergency physician with a brief introduction and overview of immunotherapy drugs and their complications.

> Patients with cancer can be immunocompromised because of their underlying malignancy as well as the medical therapies with which they are treated. Infections frequently present atypically and can be challenging to diagnose. The spectrum of infectious diseases encountered in patients receiving chemotherapy, hematopoietic stem cell transplant, and immunotherapy is broad depending on the depth of immunosuppression. Early recognition of infectious processes followed by appropriate diagnostic testing, imaging, and empiric antibiotic therapy in the emergency department are critical to providing optimal care and improving survival in this complex patient population.

> Tumor lysis syndrome (TLS) is a life-threatening oncologic emergency, characterized by a constellation of hyperkalemia, hyperuricemia, hyperphosphatemia, and hypocalcemia. The spectrum ranges from patients who are asymptomatic to those who go into cardiac arrest and die. Prompt recognition and initiation of treatment by emergency physicians are key, especially in the early stages of the syndrome. This case-based review presents an overview of the key points in pathophysiology, diagnosis, and management of TLS that are key to emergency physicians.

related to either an acute anemia or a vasoocclusive crisis. Differentiating between the two is the first step in the workup. Anemic crises must then be differentiated by the source. Vasoocclusive crises must be appropriately treated with aggressive pain management, gentle hydration, and other appropriate adjuncts. Early recognition and treatment are key in providing excellent emergency care to those with sickle cell disease.

Superior vena cava syndrome occurs from obstruction of the superior vena cava. The most common cause is malignancy. Small cell lung cancer and non-Hodgkin lymphoma are the most frequent culprits. Intravascular devices associated with thrombus are becoming more common causes. Classic symptoms include edema, plethora, and distended veins of the face, neck, and chest; shortness of breath; cough; headache; and hoarseness. Treatment in the emergency department is mostly supportive, with head elevation, oxygen, and steroids. Rarely, emergent airway issues and cerebral edema must be addressed. Definitive treatment includes radiotherapy, chemotherapy, and stenting.

Today a variety of anticoagulants and antiplatelet agents are available on the market. Given the propensity for bleeding among patients prescribed these medications, the emergency medicine physician must be equipped with a working knowledge of hemostasis, and anticoagulant and antiplatelet reversal. This article reviews strategies to address bleeding complications occurring secondary to warfarin, low-molecular-weight heparin, and direct oral anticoagulant therapy.

Emergency providers are likely to encounter patients with acute and chronic leukemias. In some cases, the first presentation to the emergency department may be for symptoms related to blast crisis and leukostasis. Making a timely diagnosis and consulting a hematologist can be life saving. Presenting symptoms are caused by complications of bone marrow infiltration and hyperleukocytosis with white blood cell counts more than 100,000. Presentations may include fatigue (anemia), bleeding (thrombocytopenia), shortness of breath, and/or neurologic symptoms owing to hyperleukocytosis and subsequent leukostasis. Treatment of symptomatic cases involves induction chemotherapy and/or leukapheresis. Asymptomatic hyperleukocytosis can be treated with hydroxyurea.

Anemia is a common condition and is diagnosed on laboratory assessment. It is defined by abnormally low hemoglobin concentration or decreased red blood cells. Several classification systems exist. Laboratory markers provide important information. Acute anemia presents with symptoms caused by acute blood loss; chronic anemia may present with worsening fatigue, dyspnea, lightheadedness, or chest pain. Specific treatments depend on the underlying anemia and causes. Iron is an alternative treatment for patients with microcytic anemia due to iron deficiency. Hyperbaric oxygen is an option for alternative rescue therapy. Most patients with chronic anemia may be discharged with follow-up if hemodynamically stable.

In 2015, The James Cancer Hospital's Emergency Department (ED) opened at The Ohio State University Wexner Medical Center's ED. Careful planning was undertaken to assure that the needs of patients with cancer would be addressed. Strong relationships between experts in hematology, oncology, and emergency medicine were built to maximize the positive impact. Ongoing reevaluation of operational needs facilitates optimal patient flow, resource use, and opportunities to build and develop new resources. The results are evident in improved patient satisfaction in the cancer ED and a much smoother flow of patients into the system.

The United States cancer population is growing and is projected to grow further. The current cancer population has a high rate of emergency department admission. Further training about oncologic emergencies may be needed and would ideally strive to care for the whole patient, including sequelae of the malignancy, progressive disease, symptom control, adverse effects of treatment, and palliative care. The James Cancer Hospital at The Ohio State University Wexner Medical Center and The University of Texas MD Anderson Cancer Center fellowship training programs in oncologic emergency medicine are described.

EMERGENCY MEDICINE
CLINICS OF NORTH AMERICA

RELATED INTEREST

Hematology/Oncology Clinics, December 2017 (Vol. 31, Issue 6)
Hematology/Oncology Emergencies
John C. Perkins and Jonathan E. Davis, *Editors*

THE CLINICS ARE NOW AVAILABLE ONLINE!
Access your subscription at:
www.theclinics.com

PROGRAM OBJECTIVE
The goal of *Emergency Medicine Clinics of North America* is to keep practicing emergency medicine physicians and emergency medicine residents up to date with current clinical practice in emergency medicine by providing timely articles reviewing the state of the art in patient care.

LEARNING OBJECTIVES
Upon completion of this activity, participants will be able to:
1. Review the rapid-fire emergency room care approach to various conditions, diseases, and syndromes
2. Recognize the latest cancer agents and their complications, as well as pediatric oncologic emergencies
3. Discuss anticoagulation reversal

ACCREDITATION
The Elsevier Office of Continuing Medical Education (EOCME) is accredited by the Accreditation Council for Continuing Medical Education (ACCME) to provide continuing medical education for physicians.

The EOCME designates this enduring material for a maximum of 15 *AMA PRA Category 1 Credit*(s)™. Physicians should claim only the credit commensurate with the extent of their participation in the activity.

All other healthcare professionals requesting continuing education credit for this enduring material will be issued a certificate of participation.

DISCLOSURE OF CONFLICTS OF INTEREST
The EOCME assesses conflict of interest with its instructors, faculty, planners, and other individuals who are in a position to control the content of CME activities. All relevant conflicts of interest that are identified are thoroughly vetted by EOCME for fair balance, scientific objectivity, and patient care recommendations. EOCME is committed to providing its learners with CME activities that promote improvements or quality in healthcare and not a specific proprietary business or a commercial interest.

The planning committee, staff, authors and editors listed below have identified no financial relationships or relationships to products or devices they or their spouse/life partner have with commercial interest related to the content of this CME activity:
Angela Irene Carrick, DO, FACOEP; Stephanie Charshafian, MD; Holly Briann Costner, DO; Matthew Davis, DO; Luca R. Delatore, MD; Sarah B. Dubbs, MD; Imad El Majzoub, MD; Geremiha Emerson, MD; Akilesh P. Honasoge, MD; Colin Kaide, MD; Alison Kemp; Alex Koyfman, MD; Stephen Y. Liang, MD, MPHS; Brit Long, MD; Amal Mattu; Katie Pfaff; Lindsey Picard, MD; Michael Porter, MD; Michael G. Purcell, MD; Daniel J. Sessions, MD; Erica M. Simon, DO, MHA; Kathleen Stephanos, MD; Matthew J. Streitz, MD; Vignesh Viswanathan; Shelly Zimmerman, DO, FACOEP.

UNAPPROVED/OFF-LABEL USE DISCLOSURE
The EOCME requires CME faculty to disclose to the participants:
1. When products or procedures being discussed are off-label, unlabelled, experimental, and/or investigational (not US Food and Drug Administration [FDA] approved); and
2. Any limitations on the information presented, such as data that are preliminary or that represent ongoing research, interim analyses, and/or unsupported opinions. Faculty may discuss information about pharmaceutical agents that is outside of FDA-approved labelling. This information is intended solely for CME and is not intended to promote off-label use of these medications. If you have any questions, contact the medical affairs department of the manufacturer for the most recent prescribing information.

TO ENROLL
To enroll in the *Emergency Medicine Clinics* Continuing Medical Education program, call customer service at 1-800-654-2452 or sign up online at http://www.theclinics.com/home/cme. The CME program is available to subscribers for an additional annual fee of $235 USD.

METHOD OF PARTICIPATION
In order to claim credit, participants must complete the following:
1. Complete enrolment as indicated above.
2. Read the activity.
3. Complete the CME Test and Evaluation. Participants must achieve a score of 70% on the test. All CME Tests and Evaluations must be completed online.

CME INQUIRIES/SPECIAL NEEDS
For all CME inquiries or special needs, please contact elsevierCME@elsevier.com.

Foreword

Hematologic and Oncologic Emergencies

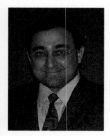

Amal Mattu, MD
Consulting Editor

In the past two decades of practicing emergency medicine, there are probably only two major conditions that seem to have markedly increased in my practice: the number of elderly patients we care for and the number of patients with cancer (in their current or past history) that we care for. The increase in elderly patients in our practice has been strongly addressed in recent years in educational conferences, textbooks and journals, and national guidelines. But cancer still seems to be a relatively ignored clinical condition in emergency medicine.

Perhaps this lack of attention is because cancer has long been considered the domain of internal medicine and oncology subspecialists. However, cancer has a tremendous influence on acute care medicine as well. Patients that have a prior history of cancer are often relatively immunocompromised and warrant more conservative treatments. Cancer has an influence on the neurologic and cardiovascular systems as well as just about every other major organ system. Patients that have ongoing cancer therapy must be evaluated for neutropenia or other hematologic abnormalities. Chemotherapy drugs can cause acute complications that force patients to the emergency department (ED), or they can interact with medications that are typically used in the ED setting.

In this issue of *Emergency Medicine Clinics of North America*, Guest Editors Drs Colin Kaide and Sarah Dubbs bring their expertise in oncology emergencies to us so we can learn how to best care for this challenging group of patients. They and their authors address a multitude of both solid organ and hematologic cancers, and they teach us about primary and secondary complications from cancer. Updates are provided on the latest chemotherapeutic agents. Complications from cancer, such as tumor lysis syndrome, hypercalcemia, superior vena cava syndrome, and hyperviscosity syndrome, among others are addressed in detail.

The editors and authors do not limit their discussion of hematologic emergencies to just cancer-related conditions. They also discuss sickle cell anemia, reversal of excess anticoagulation, and transfusion complications.

Emerg Med Clin N Am 36 (2018) xiii–xiv
https://doi.org/10.1016/j.emc.2018.05.002
0733-8627/18/© 2018 Published by Elsevier Inc.

emed.theclinics.com

This issue of *Emergency Medicine Clinics of North America* represents a mini–fellowship curriculum in oncologic emergencies for the emergency physician. This issue is a vitally important contribution to education and is certain to improve the care of this ever-growing patient population in the ED. Kudos to the Guest Editors and their authors for this excellent work.

Amal Mattu, MD
Department of Emergency Medicine
University of Maryland School of Medicine
110 South Paca Street
6th Floor, Suite 200
Baltimore, MD 21201, USA

E-mail address:
amalmattu@comcast.net

Preface

The Heme-Onc Tidal Wave: Are You Prepared?

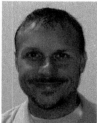 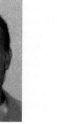

Colin G. Kaide, MD, FACEP, FAAEM   Sarah B. Dubbs, MD, FAAEM
Editors

The cancer population in the United States continues to grow and is projected to do so for the foreseeable future. Patients with hematologic and oncologic emergencies are presenting in increasing numbers to all types of emergency departments...academic, community, and rural. These patients bring a unique set of illnesses and complications, both of their primary disease and of its treatment. A functional understanding of some of the more frequently encountered emergencies in this unique population is mandatory for all practicing emergency providers.

In this issue, we chose three very different approaches in presenting hematologic and cancer-related emergencies. The first, more traditional style is a broadly encompassing article that is a more comprehensive approach to specific topics, including anticoagulation reversal, anemia and transfusion, and complications of the newest cancer therapies.

The second is a rapid-fire, case-based approach to some topics that have been very well covered in previous issues. This approach begins with a specific case or cases that illustrate the main, most important aspects of a particular heme-onc emergency. The article goes on to explain the important pathophysiology and diagnostic and treatment strategies appropriate for this specific case while also elaborating on the highlights of the diagnosis in general. We believe this format will prepare the treating clinician by providing the "nuts and bolts" necessary to care for the problem in real time without bogging the reader down with too many facts that are not pertinent for the emergency at hand.

The third section consists of 2 articles: The Dedicated Cancer Emergency Department and the Emergency Oncology Fellowship. The first article describes The Ohio State University's experience with creating the first cancer emergency department (ED) that is fully integrated into both a specialty cancer center (the James Cancer Center) and the OSU Wexner Medical Center ED. This article can provide the reader with an

Emerg Med Clin N Am 36 (2018) xv–xvi
https://doi.org/10.1016/j.emc.2018.05.001
0733-8627/18/© 2018 Published by Elsevier Inc.   emed.theclinics.com

outline of the process and experiences of creating an ED that is dedicated to patients with cancer but remains fully integrated into the bigger ED process. The second article describes the OSU emergency oncology fellowship and the MD Anderson emergency oncology fellowship as seen through the eyes of the fellows themselves. This can provide insight into what is involved in the training of an emergency physician with specific skills dedicated to treating patients with hematologic/oncologic emergencies and to elucidate why the ED doctor is the perfect candidate, uniquely qualified to treat this special population.

We hope that you find these articles informative and helpful to the clinical care of your patients, on an individual patient basis as well as for your department or hospital system. It has been a privilege to serve as guest editors for this *Emergency Medicine Clinics of North America* issue, and we are grateful to Dr Amal Mattu for the opportunity. We would also like to sincerely thank each of the authors for their contributions of time and expertise to this issue, as well as the Elsevier editorial team for their guidance and support. Please enjoy this issue of *Emergency Medicine Clinics of North America* Hematology/Oncology Emergencies! Oh, and in case of a tidal wave, this issue can be used as a floatation device!

Colin G. Kaide, MD, FACEP, FAAEM
Department of Emergency Medicine
Wexner Medical Center at
The Ohio State University
760 Prior Hall
376 West 10th Avenue
Columbus, OH 43210, USA

Sarah B. Dubbs, MD, FAAEM
Department of Emergency Medicine
University of Maryland School of Medicine
110 South Paca Street
6th Floor, Suite 200
Baltimore, MD 21201, USA

E-mail addresses:
colin.kaide@osumc.edu (C.G. Kaide)
sdubbs@som.umaryland.edu (S.B. Dubbs)

The Latest Cancer Agents and Their Complications

Sarah B. Dubbs, MD

KEYWORDS

- Cancer • Immunotherapy • Checkpoint modulators • Cancer vaccines
- Adoptive immunotherapy • CAR-T • Immune-related adverse events
- Oncologic emergency

KEY POINTS

- Cancer immunotherapy is a new class of cancer agents that leverages the immune system to combat cancer.
- The mechanisms of action are vastly different than traditional cytotoxic chemotherapy.
- Complications related to immunotherapy, termed immune-related adverse events (IRAEs) occur frequently, affect almost any organ system, but most are mild to moderate in severity and are self-limited or respond to steroids.
- Emergency physicians must be aware of IRAEs and be able to diagnose and manage them in consultation with oncologists.

INTRODUCTION

Emergency physicians have grown comfortable with diagnosing and treating the various infectious, cardiovascular, gastrointestinal, dermatologic, and other complications of traditional cytotoxic chemotherapies, but the armamentarium of cancer therapeutics available to oncologists has grown exponentially over the last decade. There is now an entirely new class of cancer therapeutics, known as cancer immunotherapy, and it works by entirely different mechanisms and has completely different complications. New drugs and new indications are being approved at a rapid pace, and it is imperative that emergency physicians become familiar with the diagnosis and management of complications associated with these drugs.

The cornerstone difference between cancer immunotherapy and traditional chemotherapy is that the primary goal of immunotherapy is to interfere with growth signals produced by cancerous cells, rather than directly destroy them (and other healthy cells

Disclosure Statement: The author reports no relationship with a commercial company that has a direct financial interest in subject matter or materials discussed in this article or with a company making a competing product.
Department of Emergency Medicine, University of Maryland School of Medicine, 110 South Paca Street, 6th Floor, Suite 200, Baltimore, MD 21201, USA
E-mail address: sdubbs@som.umaryland.edu

Emerg Med Clin N Am 36 (2018) 485–492
https://doi.org/10.1016/j.emc.2018.04.006
0733-8627/18/© 2018 Elsevier Inc. All rights reserved.

emed.theclinics.com

in the process). The mechanism by which immunotherapy achieves this goal is by enhancing antitumor immune responses of the patient's immune cells.

OVERVIEW OF IMMUNE-BASED THERAPIES

Several strategies have been developed, aimed at priming the immune system's response to tumor cells, leading to the genesis of several different immunotherapy agents. A familiarity with these modalities will enable emergency physicians to not only understand the mechanisms of action, but also to anticipate potential complications when patients undergoing immune therapy present to the emergency department.

To date, there are 3 main immunotherapeutic strategies.[1] These include nonspecific stimulation of immune reactions, active immunization to enhance antitumor reaction, and passive transfer of activated immune cells with antitumor activity. **Table 1** summarizes these methods.

Nonspecific Stimulation

Interleukin-2 (IL-2) is a T-cell growth factor that was first identified in 1980,[2] then became more widely studied in 1983 when a recombinant form was developed.[3] A landmark trial by Rosenberg and colleagues[4] was the first to document regression of advanced solid cancers using immunotherapy in people. The trial analyzed effects of IL-2 and LAK (nonspecific lymphokine-activated natural killer) cells together, but a follow-up trial[5] showed that the response was in fact due to IL-2 alone. IL-2 works by stimulating T and natural killer cells in order to act on tumor cells recognized as foreign. IL-2 was originally approved in the 1990s as monotherapy to treat metastatic renal cell cancer and metastatic melanoma. Today, treatment is approved for several other malignancies including nonsmall cell lung cancer (NSCLC) using IL-2, typically in combination with other therapies (other methods of immune therapy as well as with chemotherapy).[6]

The other subcategory of nonspecific immune system stimulation is recognized as checkpoint modulator therapy (also called checkpoint inhibitors but will be referred in this article as checkpoint modulators). To date, there are 3 mechanisms of checkpoint modulators: anticytotoxic T-lymphocyte antigen 4 (anti-CTLA-4), antiprogrammed death 1 (anti-PD-1), and antiprogrammed death ligand 1 (anti-PDL1). They differ in mechanism from IL-2; instead of stimulating the immune cells directly, these antibody drugs remove inhibitory mechanisms that are typically in place to dampen the immune response. In other words, they modulate the points that keep the immune system in check, effectively taking the brakes off of the system. Currently, available checkpoint inhibitors include ipilimumab (anti-CTLA-4), nivolumab and pembrolizumab

Table 1
Summary of methods, mechanism, and agents of cancer immunotherapy

Method	Mechanism	Agent
Nonspecific	Stimulation of effector cells Inhibition of regulatory factors ("checkpoint modulators")	IL-2 Anti-CTLA4 (ipilimumab), Anti-PD1 (nivolumab, pembrolizumab), Anti-PDL1 (atezolizumab, durvalumab)
Cancer vaccine	Active immunization to enhance antitumor reactions	Sipuleucel-T, talimogene laherparepvec
Adoptive immunotherapy	Passive transfer of activated immune cells with antitumor activity	CAR-T (tisagenlecleucel, axicabtagene ciloleucel)

(anti-PD-1), and atezolizumab and durvalumab (anti-PDL1). Each is approved for its own array of indications.

Cancer Vaccines

Cancer vaccines employ the theory that patients can be actively immunized against particular cancer antigens and generate a cellular immune response capable of combating the growth of cancer cells. The first cancer vaccine was approved in the United States in 2010; sipuleucel-T showed a modest but statistically significant improvement in overall survival in men with metastatic hormone-refractory prostate cancer.[7] This vaccine is patient specific, and is created through a process where the patient's own antigen-presenting dendritic cells are isolated from the blood and cultured with granulocyte-macrophage colony-stimulating factor, which is linked to prostatic acid phosphatase (PAP-GM-CSF). This is then infused back into the patient with the intent that the antigen-presenting dendritic cells that have been exposed to PAP-GM-CSF will stimulate the immune system T-cells to kill tumor cells that express the prostatic acid phosphatase (PAP).[7] Another cancer vaccine, called talimogene laherparepvec, is an oncolytic vaccine, and was approved in 2015 for some patients with metastatic melanoma that cannot be surgically removed.

Adoptive Immunotherapy

Adoptive immunotherapy aims to potentiate the patient's immune response to the tumor using his or her own cytotoxic T-cells. First, the patient's cells are harvested either from the tumor itself, or from the blood and genetically modified with a tumor-specific receptor, more specifically called chimeric antigen receptor T (CAR-T cell therapy). Cells with the greatest antitumor activity are assayed and selected for expansion in culture. The patient then undergoes lymphodepleting chemotherapy, followed by infusion of the replicated T-cells. The first CAR-T therapies were approved in 2017- tisagenlecleucel and axicabtagene ciloleucel.

COMPLICATIONS OF IMMUNOTHERAPY

With the mechanisms of immunotherapy action being so different from that of traditional chemotherapy, one must expect that the adverse effects and complications would be different also. In general, these adverse effects and complications are often referred to as immune-related adverse events (IRAEs). They occur as a result of overactivation of the immune system, as opposed to complications stemming from immunosuppression seen in cytotoxic chemotherapy. Because this class of medications is so new, experiential data on IRAEs are relatively limited.[8]

IRAEs have been most extensively studied in checkpoint modulators. The adverse effects and complications can potentially affect any tissue in the body, but are most prominent in systems with high cell turnover such as the gastrointestinal system, skin, endocrine glands, lungs, and liver. IRAEs occur in up to 90% of patients treated with an anti-CTLA-4 drug,[9] and 70% of those treated with a PD-1 or PD-L1 drug.[10,11] The adverse events range in severity, and tend to occur along a predictable timeline, with most occurring within 3 to 6 months of treatment initiation.[12] Most of these adverse events can be managed with corticosteroids; however, dampening the immune response may compromise gains made against the tumor.

Immune-Related Adverse Events Grading of Severity

The grading IRAE severity is based on the common terminology criteria for adverse events (CTCAEs) scale developed by the National Cancer Institute.[13] The scale ranges from 1 (mild) to 5 (death). For emergency physicians, it is not necessary to hone in on a specific score on the CTCAE, as the cutoffs for specific complaints are arbitrary. More important for all clinicians is clinical judgment rather than strictly adhering to the guidelines.[14]

Immune-Related Adverse Events by Organ Involvement

The clinical spectrum of IRAEs is summarized in **Fig. 1**.

Skin and mucosa

Vitiligo, pruritis, erythema, dry mouth, mucositis, and other dermatologic symptoms represent the most frequent IRAEs. Some case reports, although rare, have been made of Stevens Johnson syndrome/toxic epidermal necrolysis related to checkpoint modulators.

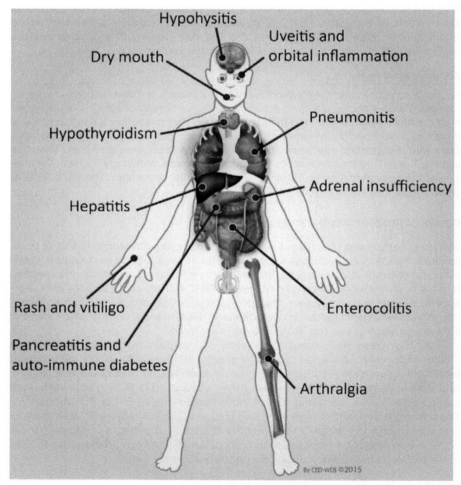

Fig. 1. Common immune-related adverse events. (*From* Michot JM, Bigenwald C, Champiat S, et al. Immune-related adverse events with immune checkpoint blockade: a comprehensive review. Eur J Cancer 2016;54:144; with permission.)

Intestinal system
Diarrhea is more common in patients taking anti-CTLA-4 therapy, occurring in about 30% of patients overall, with 10% suffering from severe (grade III-IV) diarrhea. If colitis develops (increased stool frequency and abdominal pain or colonic inflammation on imaging), a work-up for infectious causes, as well as imaging with computed tomography (CT) is recommended.[12]

Pulmonary system
A small but significant percentage of patients on immune modulators experiences immune-related pneumonitis, which can be life-threatening. Symptoms include dry cough and shortness of breath. Rales can be auscultated on examination. Advanced imaging such as a CT obtained in these patients reveals ground glass opacities and/or disseminated nodular infiltrates, especially in the lower lobes.[15] Care should be taken to also rule-out congestive heart failure or pulmonary infection.

Endocrine system
Endocrine IRAEs include thyroid dysfunction (more commonly hypothyroid than hyperthyroid)[10,16] and hypophysitis (resulting in low levels of adrenocorticotropic hormone [ACTH], thyroid stimulating hormone, follicle-stimulating hormone, luteinizing hormone, growth hormone, or prolactin). Additionally, adrenal insufficiency and diabetes mellitus can present as IRAEs.

Hepatic system
Most patients are asymptomatic and present with only elevated liver enzymes on screening to indicate immune-related hepatitis.[17] Still, viral infections with hepatitis A, B, C, and E should be investigated.

Very rare immune-related adverse events
Ophthalmic disorders Episcleritis, conjunctivitis, uveitis, and inflammation of the orbit have been reported.

Neurologic disorders Immune-mediated and inflammatory related diseases such as Guillian-Barre syndrome, aseptic meningitis, posterior reversible encephalopathy syndrome, inflammatory enteric neuropathy, and transverse myelitis have been reported in patients on anti-CTLA-4 treatment.[12]

Rheumatologic disorders Arthralgias occur in approximately 5% of patients on immune checkpoint modulators. A few cases of other rheumatologic disease such as lupus, polymyalgia rheumatic, and giant cell arteritis have been reported as well.[12]

Renal disorders Renal failure is rare but have been reported with an incidence of 1%.[15,18,19]

Hematologic disorders Autoimmune anemia, neutropenia, thrombocytopenia, and acquired hemophilia A have been reported in connection with checkpoint modulators.[14]

MANAGEMENT OF IMMUNE-RELATED ADVERSE EVENTS FOR THE EMERGENCY DEPARTMENT PHYSICIAN

The most important thing for the emergency physician to do regarding IRAEs is to first recognize and diagnose. Vigilance should also be maintained regarding life-threatening diagnoses on the differential, namely sepsis from infections, heart failure, and surgical emergencies.

Table 2
Generalized management approach to immune-related adverse events associated with immune checkpoint modulators, based on common terminology criteria for adverse events severity grade

Severity CTCAE Grade	Type of Patient Care	Steroids	Other Immunosuppressive Drugs	Immunotherapy and Subsequent Approach
1	Ambulatory	Not recommended	Not recommended	Continue
2	Ambulatory	Topical steroids or systemic steroids oral 0.5–1 mg/kg/d	Not recommended	Suspend[a] temporarily
3	Hospitalization	Systemic steroids oral or intravenously 1–2 mg/kg/d for 3 d then reduce to 1 mg/kg/d	To be considered for patients with unresolved symptoms after 3–5 d of steroid course	Suspend and discuss resumption based on risk/benefit ratio with patient
4	Hospitalization consider the intensive care unit	Systemic steroids IV methylprednisolone 1–2 mg/kg/d for 3 d and then reduce to 1 mg/kg/d	Organ specialist advised to be considered for patients with unresolved symptoms after 3–5 d of steroid course Organ specialist advised	Discontinue permanently

The overall management approach and actions to be implemented for IRAEs associated with immune checkpoint blockade, according to the CTCAE severity grade.

[a] Outside skin or endocrine disorders, where immunotherapy can be maintained.

From Michot JM, Bigenwald C, Champiat S, et al. Immune-related adverse events with immune checkpoint blockade: a comprehensive review. Eur J Cancer 2016;54:143; with permission.

Management of IRAEs is guided largely by the pharmaceutical manufacturers in conjunction with the US Food and Drug Administration, and can be found on the medication packaging and official Web site. **Table 2** displays a generalized management approach based on CTCAE severity grade. With that said, management decisions must always be made in conjunction with the patient's primary oncologist, even when the severity is mild or moderate.

SUMMARY

These latest cancer immunotherapy drugs have accelerated the ability to battle cancer. Their targeted mechanisms seem ideal, but they do come with complications. As these therapies become more widespread, emergency physicians everywhere must be aware of the immune-related adverse events that can occur, and be ready to identify and coordinate treatment.

REFERENCES

1. Rosenberg SA, Robbins PF, Phan GQ, et al. Cancer immunotherapy. In: Devita VT Jr, Lawrence TS, Rosenberg SA, editors. Cancer principles and practice of oncology. 10th edition. Philadelphia: Wolters Kluwer Health; 2015. p. 158–73.
2. Smith KA, Gilbride KJ, Favata MF. Lymphocyte activating factor promotes T-cell growth factor production by cloned murine lymphoma cells. Nature 1980;287: 853–5.
3. Rosenberg SA, Grimm EA, McGrogan M, et al. Biological activity of recombinant human interleukin-2 produced in *Escherichia coli*. Science 1984;223:1412–4.
4. Rosenberg SA, Lotze MT, Muul LM, et al. Observations on the systemic administration of autologous lymphokine-activated killer cells and recombinant interleukin-2 to patients with metastatic cancer. N Engl J Med 1985;313:1485–92.
5. Rosenberg SA, Lotze MT, Yang JC, et al. Prospective randomized trial of high-dose interleukin-2 alone or in conjunction with lymphokine-activated killer cells for the treatment of patients with advanced cancer. J Natl Cancer Inst 1993;85: 622–32.
6. Jiang T, Zhou C, Ren S. Role of IL-2 in cancer immunotherapy. Oncoimmunology 2016;5(6):e1163462.
7. Kantoff PW, Higano CS, Shore ND, et al. Sipuleucel-T immunotherapy for castration-resistant prostate cancer. N Engl J Med 2010;363:422.
8. Chen TW, Razak AR, Bedard PL, et al. A systematic review of immune-related adverse event reporting in clinical trials of immune checkpoint inhibitors. Ann Oncol 2015;26:1824–9.
9. Hodi FS, O'Day SJ, McDermott DF, et al. Improved survival with ipilimumab in patients with metastatic melanoma. N Engl J Med 2010;363:711–23.
10. Topalian SL, Hodi FS, Brahmer JR, et al. Safety, activity, and immune correlates of anti-PD-1 antibody in cancer. N Engl J Med 2012;366:2443–54.
11. Brahmer JR, Tykodi SS, Chow LQM, et al. Safety and activity of anti-PD-L1 antibody in patients with advanced cancer. N Engl J Med 2012;366:2455–65.
12. Michot JM, Bigenwald C, Champiat S, et al. Immune-related adverse events with immune checkpoint blockade: a comprehensive review. Eur J Cancer 2016;54: 139–48.
13. National Cancer Institute. Common terminology criteria for adverse events (CTCAE) v4.0. 2009. Available at: http://evs.nci.nih.gov/ftp1/CTCAE/CTCAE_4. 03_2010-06 14_QuickReference_5x7.pdf.

14. Kumar V, Chaudhary N, Garg M, et al. Current diagnosis and management of immune related adverse events (irAEs) induced by immune checkpoint inhibitor therapy. Front Pharmacol 2017;8:49.

15. Nishino M, Sholl LM, Hodi FS, et al. Anti-PD-1-related pneumonitis during cancer immunotherapy. N Engl J Med 2015;373:288–90.

16. Robert C, Schachter J, Long GV, et al. Pembrolizumab versus ipilimumab in advanced melanoma. N Engl J Med 2015;372(26):2521–32.

17. Kim KW, Ramaiya NH, Krajewski KM, et al. Ipilimumab associated hepatitis: imaging and clinicopathologic findings. Invest New Drugs 2013;31:1071–7.

18. Voskens CJ, Goldinger SM, Loquai C, et al. The price of tumor control: an analysis of rare side effects of anti-CTLA-4 therapy in metastatic melanoma from the ipilimumab network. PLoS One 2013;8:e53745.

19. Wolchok JD, Kluger H, Callahan MK, et al. Nivolumab plus ipilimumab in advanced melanoma. N Engl J Med 2013;369:122–33.

Rapid Fire: Infectious Disease Emergencies in Patients with Cancer

Stephanie Charshafian, MD[a], Stephen Y. Liang, MD, MPHS[a,b,*]

KEYWORDS

- Infections • Cancer • Neutropenic fever • Hematopoietic stem cell transplant
- Cytokine release syndrome • Emergency department

KEY POINTS

- Infections in the patients with cancer can be difficult to diagnose because of their immunocompromised state, lack of typical inflammatory signs and symptoms, and atypical clinical presentations. Fever is often the only presenting symptom.
- Emergency physicians should maintain a high index of suspicion for infection in patients with cancer seeking care in the emergency department. Timely initiation of empiric antibiotic therapy is paramount, and a low threshold for inpatient admission is advisable.
- Patients with chemotherapy-related neutropenia are at risk for common bacterial as well as fungal infections. Hematopoietic stem cell transplant patients are at risk of infection with a broader range of organisms, including bacteria, viruses, and fungi, both common and atypical.
- Cytokine release syndrome can occur in patients receiving T-cell engaging immunotherapies. Although not infectious in origin, its initial clinical presentation may be indistinguishable from infection.

Disclosure: S. Charshafian reports no conflicts of interest and no financial disclosures. S.Y. Liang reports no conflicts of interest in this work. S.Y. Liang is the recipient of a KM1 Comparative Effectiveness Research Career Development Award (KM1CA156708-01) and received support through the Clinical and Translational Science Award (CTSA) program (UL1RR024992) of the National Center for Advancing Translational Sciences as well as the Barnes-Jewish Patient Safety & Quality Career Development Program, which is funded by the Foundation for Barnes-Jewish Hospital.
[a] Division of Emergency Medicine, Washington University School of Medicine, 4523 Clayton Avenue, Campus Box 8072, St Louis, MO 63110, USA; [b] Division of Infectious Diseases, Washington University School of Medicine, 4523 Clayton Avenue, Campus Box 8051, St Louis, MO 63110, USA
* Corresponding author. 4523 Clayton Avenue, Campus Box 8051, St Louis, MO 63110.
E-mail address: syliang@wustl.edu

Emerg Med Clin N Am 36 (2018) 493–516
https://doi.org/10.1016/j.emc.2018.04.001
emed.theclinics.com

CASE 1: NEUTROPENIC FEVER

Pertinent history: a 62-year-old woman with acute lymphoblastic leukemia (ALL) undergoing chemotherapy consisting of vincristine, doxorubicin, and prednisone presents to the emergency department (ED) for a documented oral temperature of 38.3°C (100.9° F). She takes her temperature daily and has not had a fever previously. She has no history of neutropenia. Her review of systems is positive only for mild lower abdominal pain. She denies headache, neck pain, cough, dyspnea, nausea, vomiting, diarrhea, dysuria, hematuria, urinary urgency or frequency, rash, odynophagia, or tenderness along her port site.

Physical examination: temperature, 38.6°C (101.5°F); blood pressure, 135/75 mm Hg; pulse, 85 beats/min; respiration rate (RR), 14 breaths/min; oxygen saturation (SpO$_2$), 97%.

General: well appearing, no acute distress.
Oropharynx: no oropharyngeal lesions or plaques.
Neck: supple without meningismus.
Cardiovascular: regular rate and rhythm without murmurs, rubs, or gallops.
Pulmonary: lungs clear to auscultation bilaterally.
Chest: right chest port site without erythema, fluctuance, tenderness, or drainage.
Abdomen: soft, mild tenderness to palpation in the right lower abdomen without rebound or guarding; bowel sounds are present.
Skin: warm and well perfused; no rashes, erythema, or swelling.
Neurologic: awake, alert, oriented ×4, normal strength and sensation throughout.

Diagnostic testing			
WBC ($\times 10^9$/L)	2.4	BUN (mg/dL)	12
ANC (cells/µL)	370	Creatinine (mg/dL)	0.8
Hgb (g/dL)	12.2	AST (IU/L)	34
Platelets ($\times 10^9$/L)	380	ALT (IU/L)	18
Na (mEq/L)	142	Alkaline phosphatase (IU/L)	160
K (mEq/L)	3.8	Bilirubin (mg/dL)	0.7
Cl	101	CO$_2$ (mEq/L)	26

Abbreviations: ANC, absolute neutrophil count; BUN, blood urea nitrogen; Hgb, hemoglobin; WBC, white blood cell count.

Urinalysis: negative nitrites, negative leukocyte esterase; no WBCs, red blood cells, or bacteria.
Plan: obtain blood cultures (1 set from port, 1 set from peripheral venipuncture) and urine culture. Initiate empiric antibiotics for neutropenic fever. Perform computed tomography (CT) of the abdomen and pelvis.
Update: CT shows bowel wall thickening of the cecum and distal ilium without stranding or pneumatosis. Because of concern for neutropenic enterocolitis, general surgery is consulted and the patient is admitted to the oncology ward for empiric broad-spectrum antibiotics.

LEARNING POINTS: NEUTROPENIC FEVER
Introduction and Background

1. As the US population continues to expand and age, modern advances in early cancer detection and treatment have dramatically improved cancer survivorship. More

than 15 million people with a history of cancer were living in the United States alone in 2016.[1]

2. Patients with cancer are at high risk of infection because of anatomic obstruction related to tumor infiltration (eg, postobstructive pneumonia), mucosal barrier compromise caused by cytotoxic chemotherapy, and defective immunity in the context of immunosuppressive cancer therapy or hematologic malignancy.

3. Chemotherapy is a mainstay of cancer treatment, and neutropenia is a common, well-known side effect. Neutropenic fever occurs in 10% to 50% of patients with solid tumors and more than 80% of patients with hematologic malignancy undergoing chemotherapy; it carries a mortality of nearly 10%.[2–4] In 2012, more than 100,000 patients with cancer were admitted to US hospitals for neutropenia and/or its infectious complications. These neutropenia-related hospitalizations result in significant morbidity and mortality, incurring substantial medical costs.[3–5]

4. Emergency physicians play a critical role in the time-sensitive diagnosis, stabilization, and management of patients presenting to acute care with neutropenic fever and other common infectious complications of chemotherapy.

Pathology/Pathophysiology

1. Essentially all chemotherapeutic agents have immunosuppressive effects. Although different agents act on a variety of cellular functions, the common thread is that they interfere with the proliferative capacity of immune cells through bone marrow suppression,[6] the most significant side effect being neutropenia.[7]
   - The ANC reaches its nadir about 7 to 14 days after treatment and begins to return to normal levels 3 to 4 weeks after treatment.[8]

2. Hematologic malignancies and myelodysplastic syndromes resulting in bone marrow failure as well as solid organ tumors infiltrating the bone marrow also lead to neutropenia. Neutropenia is commonly defined as an ANC less than 1500 cells/μL in adults. Neutropenia can be further classified by severity:
   - Mild: ANC 1000 to 1500 cells/μL
   - Moderate: ANC 500 to 1000 cells/μL
   - Severe: ANC less than 500 cells/μL[9]
   - Profound: ANC less than 100 cells/μL[10]
     - The risk of infection is inversely proportional to the ANC. Infection is unlikely with ANC greater than 1000 cells/μL, greatly increased with ANC less than 500 cells/μL, and severely increased with ANC less than 100 to 200 cells/μL.[9]

ANC calculation

ANC = (% neutrophils + % bands) × WBC count (cells/μL)

Example: WBC = 2000 (cells/μL) and neutrophils = 10% and bands = 2%

Then ANC = 12% × 2000 (cells/μL) = 240 (cells/μL)

---

3. Infectious Disease Society of America (IDSA) and National Comprehensive Cancer Network (NCCN) guidelines define neutropenic fever as an ANC less than 500 cells/μL (or ANC <1000 cells/μL with expected decline to <500 cells/μL over the next 48 hours) and either a single oral temperature of ≥38.3°C (101.0°F) or a temperature of ≥38.0°C (100.4°F) sustained for 1 hour.[10,11]

4. Neutrophils are the first line of defense in the innate immune system and play a key role in host response to bacterial and fungal pathogens. Neutropenic patients are therefore at high risk of infection with these organisms, particularly when cytotoxic

chemotherapy compromises the integrity of mucosal barriers (ie, mucositis). Translocation of colonizing organisms across these barriers leads to invasive infection.[7]

- Common organisms encountered in neutropenic fever include gram-negative bacteria (eg, *Escherichia coli*, *Klebsiella pneumoniae*, *Pseudomonas aeruginosa*) and gram-positive bacteria (eg, *Streptococcus* spp, *Staphylococcus aureus*, coagulase-negative *Staphylococcus*, *Enterococci* spp).[12–14]
- *Candida* can cause mucosal infections (eg, oral thrush, esophagitis) as well as bloodstream and other invasive infections in the setting of chemotherapy-induced mucositis or central venous catheter infection. Invasive candidiasis is not typically encountered until after the first week of prolonged neutropenia.
- Molds (such as *Aspergillus* spp, Zygomycetes, and *Fusarium*) are most likely to cause life-threatening invasive infections after 2 or more weeks of neutropenia, and typically only in patients with profound neutropenia. In addition, patients undergoing treatment of acute myelogenous leukemia are especially susceptible to invasive mold infections.[10,15,16]

Making the Diagnosis

1. Initial and timely (within 15 minutes of triage) assessment of patients presenting with neutropenic fever to the ED should begin with[10,17]:
   - Complete blood cell count with differential and comprehensive metabolic panel (serum electrolytes, blood urea nitrogen, creatinine, hepatic transaminases, bilirubin)
   - At least 2 sets of aerobic and anaerobic blood cultures:
     ○ One set of blood cultures from each lumen of any indwelling vascular access device (eg, central venous catheter, implantable port) plus 1 peripheral venipuncture site, or
     ○ Two sets of blood cultures from different peripheral venipuncture sites
   - Fungal blood cultures:
     ○ Fungal blood cultures should be obtained in patients at significant risk for developing candidemia (eg, active chemotherapy, hematologic malignancy, solid organ or hematopoietic stem cell transplant (HSCT), patients with a central venous catheter, those receiving total parenteral nutrition)
   - Culture from other sites of suspected infection (eg, urine, sputum, wound, cerebrospinal fluid [CSF]), based on clinical suspicion.
2. Apart from fever, neutropenic patients may lack the necessary inflammatory response to manifest classic signs and symptoms of infection.
   - Erythema and induration can be mild with cellulitis, radiographic infiltrates subtle or absent in pneumonia, pyuria lacking despite a symptomatic urinary tract infection, and meningeal signs minimal if present at all in meningitis.[10]
   - Physicians should note that severely or profoundly neutropenic patients can present with suspected infection and either lack fever or be hypothermic.[17]
3. A detailed history of symptoms tailored to organ-specific infections as well as a thorough physical examination to identify subtle signs of infection should be performed, paying close attention to the skin, oropharynx, lungs, and gastrointestinal tract.
4. Unique considerations when diagnosing organ-specific infections in the setting of neutropenia:
   - Oropharyngeal infection:
     ○ White plaques are typical of oral candidiasis and are frequently asymptomatic. Painful oral ulcers or vesicles are more likely to represent infection with herpes simplex virus (HSV).[11]

- Infectious esophagitis
  - Retrosternal burning, dysphagia, and odynophagia should prompt suspicion for *Candida*, HSV, or cytomegalovirus (CMV) infection.[11] Upper endoscopy with biopsy of suspicious lesions is necessary to differentiate the cause and guide therapy.
- Sinusitis:
  - Sinus tenderness, periorbital swelling and/or cellulitis, unilateral eye tearing, or nasal erosions should prompt further evaluation. The sinuses are a common site for bacterial infection in neutropenic patients. High-risk patients (prolonged neutropenia, high-dose glucocorticoids, or graft-versus-host disease [GVHD]) are susceptible to sinusitis caused by invasive molds.[11]
  - Symptomatic patients should undergo CT of the sinuses, with a low threshold to consult an otolaryngologist and/or ophthalmologist. MRI of the orbits and brain should be performed if proptosis or cranial nerve deficits are present to evaluate for orbital abscess (**Fig. 1**) and septic cavernous sinus thrombosis.[11]
- Skin and soft tissue infection (SSTI):
  - Because of inhibition of the normal inflammatory cascade, patients with SSTI may have minimal if any erythema, warmth, induration, or purulent drainage.[10]
- Pulmonary infections:
  - Chest radiography should be obtained in any patient with respiratory symptoms. Recognize, however, that neutropenic patients with pneumonia may not show pulmonary infiltrates on plain films.[10]

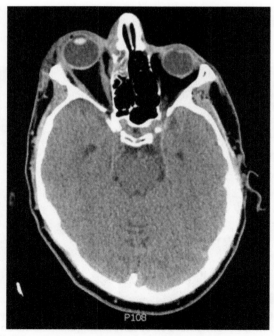

Fig. 1. Orbital cellulitis. CT showing marked proptosis of the right eye and a collection above the right orbital floor tracking from the laminal papyracea. (*From* Mahmood H, Flora H, Murphy C, et al. Retrobulbar abscess: rare complication after repair of an oroantral communication. Br J Oral Maxillofac Surg 2018;56(3). [pii:S0266-4356(18)30054-8].)

- CT of the chest may better characterize early infiltrates concerning for pneumonia.[11]
- Consider respiratory virus (including influenza) testing and urine *Legionella* antigen testing as clinically appropriate.[11,17]
- Neutropenic enterocolitis:
  - Also known as typhlitis or ileocecal syndrome, neutropenic enterocolitis is rare but potentially life threatening. Microbial invasion of the bowel wall leads to inflammation, edema, and ulceration that can progress to transmural necrosis and perforation. Untreated, multisystem organ failure and death ensue, with mortalities approaching 30% to 50%.
  - Symptoms include abdominal pain, nausea, vomiting, diarrhea, gastrointestinal hemorrhage, and peritonitis.
  - Patients with neutropenic fever and right-sided abdominal pain (the classic presentation for neutropenic enterocolitis), as well as those with neutropenia and a clinically concerning abdominal examination (eg, significant tenderness, peritoneal signs) should undergo CT of the abdomen and pelvis to rule out neutropenic enterocolitis (**Fig. 2**).[10,18,19]
- *Clostridium difficile* infection (CDI):
  - Patients presenting with unexplained, new-onset diarrhea ($\geq$3 unformed stools in 24 hours) should undergo stool testing for *C difficile*.[11,20] Recent antibiotic exposure and chemotherapy are risk factors for CDI.
  - Patients recently diagnosed with CDI (within 7 days) do not require retesting when presenting during the same episode of diarrhea.[20]
  - Patients without diarrhea should not be tested for *C difficile* because asymptomatic colonization is possible and shedding of spores may persist even after CDI treatment.[20]

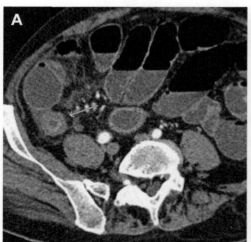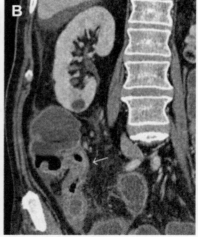

Fig. 2. (*A*) CT scan through the base of the cecum shows circumferential wall thickening of distal ileum (*arrow*) with a slight distension of surrounding small bowel and marked submucosal edema. (*B*) Coronal CT image shows the wall thickening (*arrow*) with increased edema of distal ileum and inflammatory changes in the adjacent mesenteric fat. (*From* Tiseo M, Gelsomino F, Bartolotti M, et al. Typhlitis during second-line chemotherapy with pemetrexed in non–small cell lung cancer (NSCLC): a case report. Lung Cancer 2009;65(2):251–3.)

- Urinary tract infection:
  - Obtain both a urinalysis with microscopy and urine culture in neutropenic patients with dysuria, frequency, urgency, suprapubic pain, and/or hematuria.[11]
  - Neutropenic patients with urinary tract infection may not exhibit pyuria.[10]
- Bloodstream infection:
  - Infected vascular access devices can serve as a portal of entry for bacteria or fungi into the bloodstream.
  - If inflammation is present at the site of vascular access, culture any visible drainage and obtain blood cultures from each lumen of the device.[11]
  - Mucositis predisposes patients to translocation of oropharyngeal or gut organisms across mucosal barriers leading to bloodstream infection.
- Central nervous system infection:
  - Patients with headache and/or altered mental status should undergo head CT or brain MRI, lumbar puncture (if possible), and neurology consultation.[11]
  - CSF should be sent for glucose, protein, cell count and differential, Gram stain and bacterial culture, and HSV polymerase chain reaction at a minimum.
  - Neutropenic patients with meningitis may not exhibit a pleocytosis on CSF analysis, and normal CSF profile does not rule out meningitis and should not hinder initiation of treatment in those with suspected meningitis.[10,21,22]

Treating the Patient

1. Initial empiric antibiotic therapy
   - Start empiric antibiotics early (within 1 hour) in the setting of neutropenic fever, preferably once appropriate cultures have been obtained. Timely antibiotic administration has been shown to reduce mortality.[17,23]
   - Antibiotic selection should be bactericidal and include coverage of *P aeruginosa*, accounting for local antibiotic resistance patterns and patient risk factors.
   - For patients requiring inpatient admission, initial monotherapy with an antipseudomonal beta-lactam (eg, cefepime), a carbapenem (eg, meropenem), or piperacillin-tazobactam is recommended.[10,11]
     - Additional gram-positive coverage with vancomycin or another antibiotic is not recommended as part of initial empiric therapy except in the setting of SSTI, bloodstream infection, severe pneumonia, or hemodynamic instability.
     - A combination of vancomycin plus aztreonam or clindamycin plus ciprofloxacin is appropriate for patients with a true penicillin allergy.
   - Patients already on fluoroquinolone prophylaxis should not receive a fluoroquinolone as part of empiric antibiotic therapy for neutropenic fever.[10]
2. Expanding empiric antibiotic therapy to cover antibiotic-resistant organisms
   - Oncologic patients may be at increased risk of infection with antibiotic-resistant organisms because of:
     - Increased frequency of health care exposure due to diagnostic procedures, surgery, radiation, or chemotherapy.
     - Frequent and broad exposure to antibiotics either for prophylaxis or treatment of prior infections.
   - Empiric antibiotic therapy should be modified based on previous culture-proven infection, colonization, or treatment in a hospital with high infection rates involving antibiotic-resistant organisms (**Table 1**).
3. Expanding empiric antibiotic therapy to cover fungi
   - Empiric antifungal coverage is generally reserved for high-risk patients who have had persistent fever despite 4 to 7 days of a broad-spectrum antibacterial regimen and no identified source of fever.[10]

Table 1
Additions to empiric antibiotic therapy for patients with known antibiotic-resistant organisms

Pathogen	Addition to Empiric Therapy
MRSA	Consider the addition of vancomycin, linezolid, or daptomycin[a]
VRE	Consider the addition of linezolid or daptomycin
ESBL[a]-producing gram-negative bacteria (eg, *K pneumoniae, E coli*)	Consider early use of a carbapenem
Carbapenemase-producing gram-negative bacteria (eg, Enterobacteriaceae)	Consider tigecycline or polymyxin-colistin Infectious disease consultation strongly advised

Abbreviations: ESBL, extended spectrum beta-lactamase; MRSA, methicillin-resistant *S aureus*; VRE, vancomycin-resistant enterococci.
[a] Recognize that daptomycin is inhibited by pulmonary surfactant and is therefore not an appropriate antibiotic for treating pneumonia.
Data from Freifeld AG, Bow EJ, Sepkowitz KA, et al. Infectious Diseases Society of America. Clinical practice guideline for the use of antimicrobial agents in neutropenic patients with cancer: 2010 update by the Infectious Diseases Society of America. Clin Infect Dis 2011;52(4):e56–93.

- However, patients with systemic inflammatory response syndrome (SIRS) and neutropenia may benefit from additional antifungal coverage with voriconazole, an echinocandin (eg, caspofungin), or liposomal amphotericin B, if the suspicion for fungal infection (eg, *Candida* spp, *Aspergillus* spp) is high.[10]
4. Unique considerations for tailoring empiric antibiotic therapy to organ-specific infections
   - Oropharyngeal infections and infectious esophagitis:
     - Fluconazole is considered first-line antifungal therapy for oral candidiasis and esophagitis.[11]
     - Endoscopic findings should ultimately guide treatment of *Candida*, CMV, or HSV esophagitis.[11]
   - Sinusitis:
     - Broad-spectrum antibiotics, including anaerobic coverage, should be initiated in those with concern for bacterial sinusitis.
     - Vancomycin should be added in those with concern for periorbital cellulitis (often caused by *S aureus*).
     - Liposomal amphotericin B should be added for high-risk patients with CT or MRI findings concerning for invasive fungal sinusitis to cover molds (eg, *Aspergillus*, Zygomycetes, *Mucor*).[11]
   - SSTIs:
     - Initial empiric therapy for neutropenic fever, plus early addition of vancomycin, daptomycin, or linezolid to cover broadly for gram-positive bacteria.[10,11]
   - Pulmonary infections:
     - Initial broad-spectrum coverage should consist of a beta-lactam or carbapenem plus aminoglycoside or antipseudomonal fluoroquinolone.[10,11] In severe pneumonia (hypoxia or extensive infiltrates) or if methicillin-resistant *S aureus* (MRSA) is suspected, vancomycin or linezolid should be added.[10]
     - In high-risk populations (hematologic malignancy, HSCT, GVHD), nodular or cavitary pneumonia, segmental consolidation, or ground-glass infiltrates on chest radiograph or CT should raise concern for *Aspergillus* infection.[11] Empiric antifungal therapy should be considered in this setting.

- ○ Antiviral therapy is strongly recommended for all patients with neutropenic fever and suspected or confirmed influenza, even if symptoms have been present for more than 48 hours.[11,24]
- Prospective studies demonstrating modest reductions in influenza illness duration and risk of progression to lower respiratory tract infection were conducted primarily in otherwise healthy adults. Observational studies have shown a decrease in severe clinical outcomes associated with influenza in hospitalized and elderly patients. Although there is a paucity of data addressing immunocompromised patients with influenza, these patients are likely to have prolonged viral replication and more severe disease and are likely to benefit from antiviral therapy.[25–33]
- Neutropenic enterocolitis:
  - ○ Antibiotic coverage should include gram-negative and anaerobic bacteria using piperacillin-tazobactam, a carbapenem, or combination therapy with an antipseudomonal cephalosporin plus metronidazole.[10]
  - ○ Although some patients can be managed medically, those with sepsis, peritonitis, bowel ischemia, perforation, or gastrointestinal bleeding warrant urgent surgical consultation.[10,18,19]
- *C difficile* infection:
  - ○ Oral vancomycin is preferred initial therapy to treat *C difficile* infection.[11,20]
- Urinary tract infections
  - ○ Additional antibiotic coverage beyond empiric therapy for neutropenic fever is generally not indicated until urine cultures have resulted.[11]
- Bloodstream infections:
  - ○ For patients with suspected vascular access device infection, vancomycin should be added to empiric antibiotic therapy.[10,11]
  - ○ The decision to remove an infected device frequently hinges on the infecting organism isolated in blood culture.[10] Emergent device removal in the ED should involve consultation with hematology/oncology, infectious disease, and/or the inpatient provider unless urgent source control is necessary (eg, sepsis, septic shock).
- Central nervous system infections:
  - ○ Initial empiric therapy should include an antipseudomonal antibiotic with adequate CSF penetration (eg, cefepime, ceftazidime, or meropenem), vancomycin, and ampicillin (for coverage of *Listeria monocytogenes*).[11]
  - ○ For patients with encephalitis, high-dose acyclovir should be added to empirically cover for HSV infection.[11]

5. Management of sepsis and septic shock
   - Early empiric antibiotic administration, fluid resuscitation, source control, and vasopressor therapy remain key principles of contemporary sepsis care.[34]
   - Because many patients receive glucocorticoids as part of their cancer therapy, consider adrenal axis insufficiency and the role of hydrocortisone (100 mg of hydrocortisone intravenously) in its treatment in the setting of refractory hypotension and septic shock.

6. Outpatient management of neutropenic fever
   - Current recommendations support that carefully selected patient can be considered for outpatient oral therapy. These patients should still receive antibiotics within 1 hour of ED presentation and be monitored for ≥ 4 hours. In the ED setting, this decision should be made in conjunction with the patient's oncologist as well as taking into consideration the psychosocial considerations outlined in the NCCN guidelines (discussed later).[17]

- For patients not requiring inpatient admission, empiric oral antibiotic therapy comprising ciprofloxacin (or levofloxacin) plus amoxicillin-clavulanate (or clindamycin if penicillin allergic) is recommended.[10,11,17] Several risk scores and professional criteria exist to evaluate patients with neutropenic fever. None have been rigorously studied in the ED. In past retrospective studies, all patients were either admitted or discharged after a period of inpatient monitoring for clinical stability or improvement.
  - As with all risk scoring systems, these criteria do not take the place of clinical judgment. If a patient does not seem low risk for outpatient therapy based on clinical judgment, these scoring systems should not be applied, and patients should be admitted.
  - Patients with known antibiotic-resistant organisms (including fluoroquinolone and beta-lactam coresistance) and those already taking prophylactic fluoroquinolones should be treated as inpatients. In addition, patients undergoing induction chemotherapy for acute leukemia, or patients undergoing HSCT, are unlikely to be appropriate candidates for outpatient therapy.[10,17]
- Multinational Association for Supportive Care in Cancer (MASCC) risk index score:
  - Scoring system derived to identify patients at low risk for poor outcomes (**Box 1**).

Box 1
Multinational Association for Supportive Care in Cancer risk index scoring criteria

Characteristic	Weight
Burden of Febrile Neutropenia	
No or mild symptoms	+5
Moderate symptoms	+3
Severe symptoms	+0
Hypotension	
Systolic blood pressure ≥90 mm Hg	+5
Systolic blood pressure <90 mm Hg	+0
Active COPD	
No	+4
Yes	+0
Cancer Characteristics	
Solid tumor	+4
Hematologic malignancy without prior fungal infection	+4
Hematologic malignancy with prior fungal infection	+0
Dehydration Requiring Parenteral Fluids	
No	+3
Yes	+0
Status at Fever Onset	
Outpatient	+3
Inpatient	+0
Age	
<60 y	+2
≥60 y	+0

≥21, low risk; <21, high risk; maximum, 26.
Abbreviation: COPD, chronic obstructive pulmonary disease.

Data from Klastersky J, Paesmans M, Rubenstein EB, et al. The Multinational Association for Supportive Care in Cancer risk index: a multinational scoring system for identifying low-risk febrile neutropenic cancer patients. J Clin Oncol 2000;18(16):3038–51.

- ○ MASCC scores of $\geq$21 identified low-risk patients with a sensitivity of 71%, specificity of 68%, and positive predictive value of 91%.[35]
- ○ Several studies have validated the usefulness of the MASCC score as a predictor of poor outcome in different populations,[36–40] although some have demonstrated poor sensitivity to predict complications in febrile neutropenia.[40–43]
- ○ Mixed results exist on the MASCC score's ability to identify appropriate candidates for oral antibiotic therapy and early discharge from the hospital after a period of observation.[40,42,44–46] IDSA guidelines recommend that patients with high-risk MASCC scores be admitted for empiric antibiotic therapy, whereas carefully selected patients with low-risk MASCC scores can be considered for outpatient and/or oral antibiotic therapy.[10]
- Clinical Index of Stable Febrile Neutropenia (CISNE) score:
  - ○ Scoring system derived to evaluate outpatients with solid tumors with febrile neutropenia at low risk of serious complications and therefore identify a group of patients potentially suitable for home treatment (**Table 2**). Low-risk patients had 0% mortality and 1.1% complication rate.[41,47]
  - ○ The CISNE score has been prospectively validated and shown to outperform the MASCC score.[43,47]
- IDSA clinical practice guidelines:
  - ○ Criteria to identify low-risk patients for oral antibiotic therapy and high-risk patients for intravenous antibiotics and inpatient admission[10] (**Table 3**).

Table 2	
Clinical Index of Stable Febrile Neutropenia score	
Characteristic	**Weight**
ECOG Performance Status	
<2	+0
$\geq$2	+2
Stress-induced Hyperglycemia	
No	+0
Yes	+2
COPD	
No	+0
Yes	+1
Chronic Cardiovascular Disease	
No	+0
Yes	+1
Mucositis	
Grade <2	+0
Grade $\geq$2	+1
Monocytes	
$\geq$200/μL	+0
<200/μL	+1

Low risk, 0; intermediate risk, 1–2; high risk, $\geq$3.

Abbreviation: ECOG, Eastern Cooperative Oncology Group.

Data from Carmona-Bayonas A, Jiménez-Fonseca P, Virizuela Echaburu J, et al. Prediction of serious complications in patients with seemingly stable febrile neutropenia: validation of the clinical index of stable febrile neutropenia in a prospective cohort of patients from the FINITE study. J Clin Oncol 2015;33(5):465–71.

Table 3
Infectious Disease Society of America criteria for low-risk and high-risk febrile neutropenia

Low-Risk Criteria	High-Risk Criteria
Anticipated brief (<7 d) neutropenia	Prolonged and profound neutropenia (<100 cells/µL for >7 d)
Clinically stable	Hemodynamic instability
No medical comorbidities	COPD
	Poor functional status
	Advanced age
	Pneumonia, pulmonary infiltrate, or hypoxemia
	Altered mental state
	Gastrointestinal symptoms
	Mucositis interfering with swallowing
	Indwelling catheter infection
	Uncontrolled pain
	Uncontrolled cancer
	Hepatic or renal insufficiency

Data from Freifeld AG, Bow EJ, Sepkowitz KA, et al. Infectious Diseases Society of America. Clinical practice guideline for the use of antimicrobial agents in neutropenic patients with cancer: 2010 update by the Infectious Diseases Society of America. Clin Infect Dis 2011;52(4):e56–93.

- NCCN clinical practice guidelines:
  - Criteria developed to identify patients that can be considered for outpatient therapy[11] (**Table 4**).

CASE CONCLUSION

On hospital day 2, the patient developed worsening abdominal pain and peritonitis. She was taken to the operating room and found to have a nonviable cecum. She

Table 4
National Comprehensive Cancer Network guidelines for outpatient therapy for febrile neutropenia

High-Risk Criteria	Low-Risk Criteria	Outpatient Criteria
Anticipated prolonged severe neutropenia	Anticipated short duration of severe neutropenia (≤100 cells/µL for <7 d)	No critical laboratory results on screening tests
Pneumonia or other complex infection	No comorbid illnesses requiring inpatient management	24-h home caregiver available
Clinically unstable	ECOG 0–1	Home telephone
Significant comorbidity	Outpatient status at time of fever onset	<1 h from appropriate medical care
Mucositis grade 3 or 4	MASCC low risk (≥21)	Access to emergency facilities
Inpatient status at time of fever onset	No hepatic (5× upper limit transaminases) or renal (CrCl <30) insufficiency	Adequate home environment
MASCC high risk (<21)		Patient consent
Hepatic or renal insufficiency		
Allogenic HSCT		
Alemtuzumab therapy		
Uncontrolled or progressive cancer		

Patients can be considered for outpatient therapy if they meet none of the high-risk, most of the low-risk, and all of the outpatient criteria.

Abbreviation: CrCl, creatinine clearance.

Data from Baden LR, Swaminathan S, Angarone M, et al. Prevention and treatment of cancer-related infections, version 2.2016, NCCN clinical practice guidelines in Oncology. J Natl Compr Canc Netw 2016;14(7):882–913.

underwent resection of her distal ileum and right hemicolon with the creation of an ileostomy. She remained hospitalized for 10 days and completed a 7-day course of piperacillin-tazobactam. She returned for reanastomosis on completion of chemotherapy with an uncomplicated postoperative course.

CASE 2: FEVER IN A HEMATOPOIETIC STEM CELL TRANSPLANT PATIENT

Pertinent history: several years later, our patient from Case 1 is diagnosed with recurrent ALL. She underwent HSCT 6 weeks ago and presents to the ED with a fever of 38.1° C (100.6° F) and a 1-week history of progressive, nonproductive cough. She denies chest pain, hemoptysis, or dyspnea.

Physical examination: temperature, 38.1° C (100.6° F); blood pressure, 135/75 mm Hg; pulse 86 beats/min; RR, 18 breaths/min; Spo$_2$, 96%.

General: well appearing, no acute distress.
Oropharynx: no oropharyngeal lesions or plaques.
Cardiovascular: regular rate and rhythm without murmurs, rubs, or gallops.
Pulmonary: no respiratory distress. Auscultation reveals mild fine, dry crackles in the right mid and upper lung fields.
Chest: right chest port without erythema, warmth, fluctuance, tenderness, or drainage.
Abdomen: soft, nontender to palpation, no rebound or guarding.
Skin: warm and well perfused; no rashes, erythema, or swelling.
Neurologic: awake, alert, oriented ×4, normal strength and sensation throughout.

Diagnostic testing: ANC, 160 cells/μL. All other tests are unremarkable.
Chest radiograph: no pulmonary infiltrates, nodules, or consolidation.
Plan: obtain blood cultures. Initiate empiric antibiotics for neutropenic fever (cefepime). Order respiratory virus testing (including influenza). Perform CT of the chest.
Update: respiratory virus testing is negative. Chest CT shows ground-glass infiltrates with a 1.6-cm nodule in the right upper lobe. Infectious disease is consulted with recommendations to start empiric voriconazole in addition to cefepime and admit to the oncology service for further care.

LEARNING POINTS: FEVER IN THE HEMATOPOIETIC STEM CELL TRANSPLANT PATIENT
Introduction and Background

With the use of HSCT to treat hematologic and solid tumor malignancies comes an increased risk of common and atypical infections. Several factors influence an individual's risk of infection, including underlying patient comorbidities, stem cell source, conditioning regimen, immunosuppression regimen, and history of post-HSCT complications (particularly GVHD).[48]

Pathology/Pathophysiology

1. The risk of infection after HSCT varies across time. Before HSCT, the recipient undergoes a conditioning regimen, which prepares the bone marrow for engraftment and virtually eliminates the endogenous immune system, rendering the patient susceptible to a host of infections until the patient's immune system reconstitutes postengraftment.[49]
2. GVHD can significantly delay a patient's immune reconstitution, prolonging the risk for infection. Chronic immunosuppression (eg, glucocorticoids) to treat GVHD further compounds this risk.[49,50]

- Human leukocyte antigen (HLA)–mismatched or HLA-matched unrelated donors have a greater risk of infectious complications compared with HLA-matched related donor transplants because of higher incidence of GVHD.[49]

Making the Diagnosis

1. HSCT patients are prone to severe and atypical infections because of the effects of immunosuppression on both myeloid and lymphoid immune cell lineages.
   - Bacterial infections
     - Early after HSCT, bacterial infections associated with neutropenia, vascular access devices, and mucositis are common.[48,49]
     - Later, the risk for bacterial infection depends on the severity of GVHD and degree of immunosuppression (particularly with glucocorticoids) required to treat GVHD. HSCT patients have an increased risk of infection with encapsulated organisms (*Streptococcus pneumoniae*, *Haemophilus influenzae*, *Neisseria meningitidis*).[48,49]
   - Viral infections
     - Viral infections are common and can cause severe illness.
     - Several herpesviruses can cause clinically important infections, most notably CMV.[48,49] CMV reactivation can manifest as pneumonitis, colitis, retinitis, hepatitis, or encephalitis.[48] HSV and varicella zoster virus (VZV) can cause both localized as well as disseminated infection.[48]
     - Respiratory viruses can cause disease at any time but tend to follow seasonal patterns as in the general population. Infections frequently progress to pneumonia with rates as high as 35%, with a mortality as high as 30%. CT is more sensitive compared with chest radiography for diagnosis of pneumonia in this population. Caution is advised when diagnosing viral pneumonia, because documented viral infection does not exclude bacterial or fungal infection.[48]
   - Fungal infections
     - *Aspergillus* is the most common mold species encountered in HSCT patients.[48] Pulmonary aspergillosis can present with nodular infiltrates, cavitary lesions, segmental consolidation, or ground-glass opacities on chest imaging.
     - Infections involving yeast, primarily *Candida* spp, include oral candidiasis, esophagitis, candidemia, and hepatosplenic (chronic) infection.[48] Candidemic patients are likely to present with fever and SIRS/sepsis.[48]
     - *Pneumocystis jiroveci* (previously *Pneumocystis carinii*) infection should be considered in patients with pneumonia not taking prophylaxis (eg, trimethoprim-sulfamethoxazole), particularly in the setting of GVHD and during periods of lymphopenia.[48]
2. Infection risk caused by obliteration and reconstitution of the immune system after HSCT follows a characteristic and predictable timeline (**Fig. 3**).[48–50]
   - Pretransplant period
     - Period before infusion of stem cells.
     - Low risk of infection, which depends on underlying patient comorbidity and existing immunosuppressive therapy.[49,50]
     - Most common infections include SSTIs, oral mucosal infections, and urinary tract infections.[49]
   - Preengraftment period
     - Period from infusion of stem cells (day 0) until marrow engraftment.
     - Infection risk is related to neutropenia, mucosal barrier breakdown (mucositis), and invasive catheters, as seen in the case of neutropenic fever.

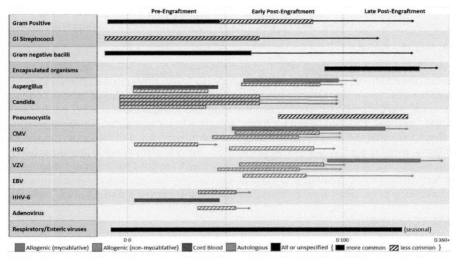

Fig. 3. Infection timeline after HSCT for most common pathogens. EBV, Epstein-Barr virus; GI, gastrointestinal; HHV, human herpesvirus. (*Data from* Refs.[48–50])

- ○ Innate immunity is the first to recover (neutrophils and epithelial barriers) 2 to 3 weeks after infusion. If engraftment is delayed, patients can have prolonged neutropenia, which places the patient at greater risk of invasive fungal infections (eg, *Candida* spp, *Aspergillus* spp).[49]
- Early postengraftment period
  - ○ Period from marrow engraftment until day 100 with early immune reconstitution.
  - ○ Impaired T-cell function leads to poor cell-mediated immunity.
  - ○ Viral infections are common during this period.
- Late postengraftment period
  - ○ Period begins around day 100 after stem cell infusion.
  - ○ Patients without development of GVHD typically regain reasonable immunity within 1 to 2 years. It takes months for the restoration of adequate B cells and CD8 T cells. CD4 T cells may remain inadequate for years, especially in older patients with less thymic reserve.
  - ○ Humoral defects lead to risk of infections with encapsulated organisms, especially of the respiratory tract, as well as viral infections, for at least 1 year.[49,50]
3. GVHD
   - Development of chronic GVHD can significantly delay restoration of normal immune function, particularly cell-mediated and humoral immunity. This can prolong the timeline for risk of infection.[49]
   - Patients with GVHD are extremely vulnerable to infectious complications because of immunosuppression from the disease process itself as well as its treatment (additional immunosuppression with glucocorticoids).[49]
     - ○ Profound immunosuppression predisposes patients with GVHD to a range of fungal (*Aspergillus* spp, *Zygomycetes*, *P jiroveci*), viral (eg, CMV, VZV), and bacterial infections.[49]
4. Post-HSCT patients, regardless of neutropenia, are functionally immunosuppressed. Any patient presenting with fever or infectious symptoms should undergo

a thorough history and physical examination, targeted imaging based on symptoms, basic laboratory testing, and microbiological cultures as clinically indicated.

Treating the Patient

The initial ED management of HSCT patients presenting with fever is no different than that of other patients with cancer with neutropenic fever, although the differential diagnosis for infection is significantly broader. HSCT patients presenting with fever should be rapidly started on broad-spectrum empiric antibiotics. Consider adding empiric antifungal coverage if the suspicion for fungal infection (eg, *Aspergillus*, *Candida*) is high.

Recognize that the diagnosis and targeted therapy for many of the opportunistic infections encountered in the HSCT population are not completed in the emergency setting. Emergency physicians should have a low threshold for inpatient admission for further diagnostic testing, and consultation with infectious disease and hematology/oncology specialists is recommended early in the care of these complex patients.

CASE CONCLUSION

The patient was continued on cefepime and voriconazole. The next morning, she underwent bronchoscopy with biopsy of the pulmonary nodule. Blood cultures remained no growth. Histopathology of lung nodule revealed hyphae and tissue culture eventually grew *Aspergillus fumigatus* on incubation day 6. Cefepime was discontinued and the patient was discharged on hospital day 10 to complete a prolonged course of voriconazole for pulmonary aspergillosis.

CASE 3: FEVER IN AN ONCOLOGY PATIENT RECEIVING IMMUNOTHERAPY

Pertinent history: our patient returns now with relapsed ALL, diagnosed 2 months ago. She is currently receiving immunotherapy with blinatumomab, a bispecific T cell–enhancing (BiTE) antibody. Treatment was initiated 16 days ago and she was discharged from the oncology ward on continuous home infusion 2 days ago. She presents to the ED for fever to 39.2°C (102.6°F). A review of systems is notable for dyspnea, malaise, and lethargy.

Physical examination: temperature, 39.3°C (102.7°F); blood pressure, 88/65 mm Hg; pulse, 110 beats/min; RR, 22 breaths/min; Spo$_2$, 87%.

General: appears lethargic with generalized weakness.
Cardiovascular: rapid rate, regular rhythm without murmurs, rubs, or gallops.
Pulmonary: mild tachypnea. Lungs clear to auscultation.
Chest: right chest port without erythema, warmth, fluctuance, tenderness, or drainage. Current infusion of medication (blinatumomab) via port.
Abdomen: soft, nontender to palpation, no rebound or guarding.
Skin: delayed capillary refill. No rashes, erythema, or mottling.
Neurologic: awake, alert, oriented ×4, nonfocal sensory and motor examination.

Diagnostic testing			
WBC (×10^9/L)	3.8	BUN (mg/dL)	12
ANC (cells/μL)	400	Creatinine (mg/dL)	0.8
Hgb (g/L)	9.8	AST (IU/L)	78
Platelets (×10^9/L)	480	ALT (IU/L)	60
Lactate (mmol/L)	3.2	Alkaline phosphatase (IU/L)	160
CO$_2$ (mEq/L)	19	Bilirubin (mg/dL)	1.1

Chest radiography: no pulmonary infiltrates, nodules, or consolidation.

Plan: stop infusion of blinatumomab. Obtain blood cultures. Resuscitate with parenteral fluids and monitor blood pressure response. Administer empiric antibiotics for neutropenic fever. Consult infectious disease and hematology/oncology. Admit to the intensive care unit (ICU).

Update: hematology/oncology raises the concern for cytokine release syndrome (CRS), recommends administration of dexamethasone in the ED, and agrees with the plan for ICU admission. Infectious disease agrees with empiric antibiotic therapy for neutropenic fever. The patient transiently responds to fluids but ultimately requires low-dose norepinephrine to maintain a mean arterial pressure greater than 60 mm Hg. She is transferred to the ICU shortly thereafter.

LEARNING POINTS: FEVER IN ONCOLOGY PATIENTS RECEIVING IMMUNOTHERAPY
Introduction and Background

Immunotherapies, such as monoclonal antibodies and chimeric antigen receptor (CAR) T-cell therapies, are an evolving class of medications used to treat cancers and other conditions, including both solid tumors and hematologic malignancies. Although there are several currently in use, there are a large number undergoing development or testing in clinical trials.[51]

Pathology/Pathophysiology

Monoclonal antibodies work by boosting the host immune response to cancer cells, blocking the growth or spread of cancer cells, or targeting immune checkpoints.[52] CARs allow major histocompatibility complex independent activation of cytotoxic T cells to target specific tumor antigens.[51,53]

1. Side effects of these medications can generally be grouped into 2 classes: autoimmune toxicity and cytokine-mediated toxicity.[53]
   - Autoimmune toxicity
     - Monoclonal antibodies, notably immune checkpoint inhibitors, can have adverse effects caused by general immune enhancement, termed immune-related adverse events (irAEs). These are common side effects and although most are mild and easily managed, they can also become life threatening. irAEs typically occur weeks to months after infusion (**Table 5**) and are treated with glucocorticoids.[52]
   - Cytokine-medicated toxicity
     - T cell–engaging immunotherapies, such as CARs or BiTE antibodies, can cause CRS. CRS is a potentially fatal condition caused by the nonphysiologic activation of T cells and subsequent release of inflammatory cytokines.[51,53]

Making the Diagnosis

CRS typically begins within 14 days of initiation of therapy.[54] Although most patients develop CRS within their hospitalization treatment periods, patients who are discharged home can also develop this syndrome and present to the ED. Many of the clinical features of CRS overlap with that of macrophage activation syndrome/hemophagocytic lymphohistiocytosis. Patients develop a systemic inflammatory response as well as increased levels of inflammatory markers, with fever often being the first sign. CRS can be self-limiting, needing only supportive care, or progress to life-threatening inflammation requiring immunosuppression (**Table 6**).[53,54] Significant overlap exists among the symptoms of CRS, neutropenic fever, and sepsis. Patients at risk for CRS are often likewise at risk for infection.[53] Emergency physicians

Table 5
Immune-related adverse events caused by immune checkpoint inhibitors

Organ System	Effects	Timing after Immunotherapy (wk)
Dermatologic	Rash (maculopapular), pruritus, vitiligo, blisters, SJS/TEN	3–6
Gastrointestinal	Diarrhea, colitis, intestinal perforation	5
Hepatic	Transaminitis, hyperbilirubinemia, fatigue, nausea, jaundice, fever, change in stool or urine color, pruritus, icterus, hepatomegaly	6–14
Endocrine	Hypopituitarism with or without hypophysitis, adrenal insufficiency, hyperthyroid/hypothyroid, gonadal hypofunction	7 and on
Other	Meningitis, uveitis, pneumonitis, pancreatitis, pericarditis, myocarditis, nephritis, angiopathies, hemolysis, thrombocytopenia	—

Abbreviations: SJS, Stevens–Johnson syndrome; TEN, toxic epidermal necrolysis.
Data from Caruana I, Diaconu I, Dotti G. From monoclonal antibodies to chimeric antigen receptors for the treatment of human malignancies. Semin Oncol 2014;41(5):661–6.

must recognize this fact, maintain a broad differential diagnosis, and treat patients accordingly.

No universal grading system exists for CRS, although the most widely accepted system used by the National Cancer Institute is summarized in **Table 7**.[39] Neurologic toxicity may be part of the spectrum of CRS but is not included in this scoring system.[53–57]

Treating the Patient

1. Treatment of CRS is aimed at supportive management and the inhibition of inflammatory cytokines.
2. Two medications are currently in use to treat CRS: glucocorticoids and tocilizumab, an interleukin-6 inhibitor. Although activation of the immune system causes CRS, it

Table 6
Signs and symptoms of cytokine release syndrome

Organ Systems	Signs and Symptoms
Constitutional	Fever, malaise, fatigue, myalgias, arthralgias, anorexia
Dermatologic	Rash
Cardiovascular	Tachycardia, wide pulse pressure, hypotension, increased cardiac output, cardiomyopathy
Pulmonary	Tachypnea, hypoxemia, acute respiratory distress syndrome
Gastrointestinal	Nausea, vomiting, diarrhea
Hepatic	Transaminitis, hyperbilirubinemia
Renal	Azotemia
Vascular	Increased D-dimer level, hypofibrinogenemia, coagulopathy, bleeding, disseminated intravascular coagulation
Neurologic	Headache, altered mental status, confusion, delirium, aphasia, hallucinations, tremor, dysmetria, seizures

Data from Brudno JN, Kochenderfer JN. Toxicities of chimeric antigen receptor T cells: recognition and management. Blood 2016;127(26):3321–30.

is also what gives these therapies their antitumor effects. For this reason, the goal of treatment is to limit life-threatening side effects of CRS while attempting to maintain antitumor effects.[48]

- Treatment of CRS related to CAR T-cell therapies:
  - The mainstay of therapy for CRS related to CAR T-cell therapies is tocilizumab.[54]
  - One treatment algorithm proposes therapy based on CRS grade and patient factors[53]:
    - Grade 1: supportive care
    - Grade 2: supportive care ± tocilizumab
    - Grade 3 or 4: supportive care + tocilizumab
- Treatment of CRS related to BiTE antibodies:
  - Pausing the infusion (the only approved BiTE antibody is administered via continuous infusion, which the patients go home on) ± administration of dexamethasone is the mainstay of treatment of CRS related to blinatumomab.[54]

3. All patients with suspected CRS should be admitted to the hospital, and those with severe symptoms should be admitted to the ICU.
4. Many institutions and/or oncology centers have their own protocols for when to administer immunosuppressants for CRS or what agent should be used. Hematology/oncology should be involved immediately in any patient presenting to the ED with suspected CRS.
5. It is often prudent to start immediate antibiotics for presumed infection in patients with febrile neutropenia, severe illness, or other infectious symptoms, even if CRS is the suspected cause, because CRS and infection cannot be differentiated based on symptoms. Infectious disease should be involved early and often.

CASE CONCLUSION

Overnight in the ICU, our patient began to show signs of hypoperfusion. Echocardiography demonstrated global cardiomyopathy with a left ventricular ejection fraction of 35%. Inotropic support was added. By the next afternoon, her fever had resolved, and

Table 7
Grading of cytokine release syndrome

Grade	Toxicity	Examples
1	Symptoms are not life threatening and require symptomatic treatment only	Fever, nausea, fatigue, headache, myalgias, malaise
2	Symptoms require and respond to moderate intervention	Oxygen requirement <40%, hypotension responsive to fluids or low-dose vasopressor, grade 2 organ toxicity[a]
3	Symptoms require and respond to aggressive intervention	Oxygen requirement ≥40%, hypotension requiring high-dose[b] or multiple vasopressors, grade 3 organ toxicity,[a] grade 4 transaminitis[a]
4	Life-threatening symptoms	Requirement for ventilatory support, grade 4 organ toxicity[a] (excluding transaminitis)
5	Death	—

[a] Grading according to the Common Terminology Criteria for Adverse Events.
[b] High-dose vasopressors: norepinephrine ≥ 20 µg/kg/min, dopamine ≥ 10 µg/kg/min, phenylephrine ≥ 200 µg/kg/min, epinephrine ≥ 10 µg/kg/min.
Data from Lee DW, Gardner R, Porter DL, et al. Current concepts in the diagnosis and management of cytokine release syndrome. Blood 2014;124(2):188–95.

Box 2
Pattern recognition

- Fever + neutropenia + clinically stable: empiric antibiotics (antipseudomonal beta-lactam [eg, cefepime], a carbapenem [eg, meropenem], or piperacillin-tazobactam)
- Neutropenic fever + SIRS: add antifungal coverage
- Neutropenic fever + hemodynamic instability: go broad-spectrum. Consider adrenal axis insufficiency
- Neutropenia + abdominal pain: neutropenic enterocolitis (typhlitis)
- Fever and/or SIRS + immunotherapy (T-cell engaging): consider CRS
- GVHD = very immunocompromised

---

she required less and less cardiovascular support. Blood cultures returned no growth at 48 hours and antibiotics were discontinued because her symptoms were thought to be related to CRS. She was discharged on hospital day 5. Outpatient follow-up showed resolution of her cardiomyopathy and she is scheduled to resume blinatumomab.

DISCUSSION

In all 3 cases, our patient was immunocompromised and at risk for infection, but for different reasons. Consequently, the differential diagnosis for infection varied widely based on cancer therapy. Patients with chemotherapy-related neutropenia are at risk for common bacterial as well as fungal infections. The differential diagnosis for infection in the HSCT population is wide-ranging. Because of significant immunosuppression and potential for GVHD, HSCT patients are at risk for a broader range of organisms, including bacteria, viruses, and fungi, both common and atypical. Patients receiving T cell–engaging immunotherapies are at risk of neutropenia (and the infections that accompany this) as well as CRS. Although CRS is not infectious in origin, its presentation is indistinguishable from infection. Emergency physicians caring for patients receiving cancer immunotherapy must be aware of this phenomenon, because treatment of infection alone does not improve the patient's clinical status.

Emergency physicians should maintain a high index of suspicion for infection in patients with cancer seeking care in the ED. Atypical presentations abound, and fever is often the only presenting symptom. Initial evaluation should include basic laboratory testing, microbiological cultures, and appropriate imaging. Timely initiation of empiric antibiotic therapy in the ED is paramount to reducing mortality, particularly in critical illness. A low threshold for inpatient admission is advisable, particularly for significantly immunocompromised patients with cancer (eg, severe, profound, or prolonged neutropenia; HSCT; GVHD). Early involvement of hematology/oncology and infectious disease specialists in the care of these complex patients helps guide empiric antibiotic therapy, diagnostic evaluation, and definitive care (**Box 2**).

REFERENCES

1. Miller KD, Siegel RL, Lin CC, et al. Cancer treatment and survivorship statistics, 2016. CA Cancer J Clin 2016;66(4):271–89.
2. Klastersky J. Management of fever in neutropenic patients with different risks of complications. Clin Infect Dis 2004;39(Suppl 1):S32–7.

3. Dulisse B, Li X, Gayle JA, et al. A retrospective study of the clinical and economic burden during hospitalizations among cancer patients with febrile neutropenia. J Med Econ 2013;16(6):720–35.

4. Kuderer NM, Dale DC, Crawford J, et al. Mortality, morbidity, and cost associated with febrile neutropenia in adult cancer patients. Cancer 2006;106(10):2258–66.

5. Tai E, Guy GP, Dunbar A, et al. Cost of cancer-related neutropenia or fever hospitalizations, United States, 2012. J Oncol Pract 2017;13(6):e552–61.

6. Harris J, Sengar D, Stewart T, et al. The effect of immunosuppressive chemotherapy on immune function in patients with malignant disease. Cancer 1976; 37(2 Suppl):1058–69.

7. Crawford J, Dale DC, Lyman GH. Chemotherapy-induced neutropenia: risks, consequences, and new directions for its management. Cancer 2004;100(2): 228–37.

8. Neutropenia. Cancer.Net. 2017. Available at: https://www.cancer.net/navigating-cancer-care/side-effects/neutropenia. Accessed December 14, 2017.

9. Boxer LA. How to approach neutropenia. Hematology Am Soc Hematol Educ Program 2012;2012:174–82.

10. Freifeld AG, Bow EJ, Sepkowitz KA, et al, Infectious Diseases Society of America. Clinical practice guideline for the use of antimicrobial agents in neutropenic patients with cancer: 2010 update by the Infectious Diseases Society of America. Clin Infect Dis 2011;52(4):e56–93.

11. Baden LR, Swaminathan S, Angarone M, et al. Prevention and treatment of cancer-related infections, version 2.2016, NCCN clinical practice guidelines in oncology. J Natl Compr Canc Netw 2016;14(7):882–913.

12. Yadegarynia D, Fatemi A, Mahdizadeh M, et al. Current spectrum of bacterial infections in patients with nosocomial fever and neutropenia. Caspian J Intern Med 2013;4(3):698–701.

13. Mandal PK, Maji SK, Dolai TK, et al. Micro-organisms associated with febrile neutropenia in patients with haematological malignancies in a tertiary care hospital in eastern India. Indian J Hematol Blood Transfus 2015;31(1):46–50.

14. Kanamaru A, Tatsumi Y. Microbiological data for patients with febrile neutropenia. Clin Infect Dis 2004;39(Suppl 1):S7–10.

15. Ramphal R. Changes in the etiology of bacteremia in febrile neutropenic patients and the susceptibilities of the currently isolated pathogens. Clin Infect Dis 2004; 39(Suppl 1):S25–31.

16. Portugal RD, Garnica M, Nucci M. Index to predict invasive mold infection in high-risk neutropenic patients based on the area over the neutrophil curve. J Clin Oncol 2009;27(23):3849–54.

17. Taplitz RA, Kennedy EB, Bow EJ, et al. Outpatient management of fever and neutropenia in adults treated for malignancy: American Society of Clinical Oncology and Infectious Diseases Society of America clinical practice guideline update. J Clin Oncol 2018. https://doi.org/10.1200/JCO.2017.77.6211.

18. Cloutier RL. Neutropenic enterocolitis. Emerg Med Clin North Am 2009;27(3): 415–22.

19. Ullery BW, Pieracci FM, Rodney JR, et al. Neutropenic enterocolitis. Surg Infect (Larchmt) 2009;10(3):307–14.

20. McDonald LC, Gerding DN, Johnson S, et al. Clinical practice guidelines for *Clostridium difficile* infection in adults and children: 2017 update by the Infectious Diseases Society of America (IDSA) and Society for Healthcare Epidemiology of America (SHEA). Clin Infect Dis 2018. https://doi.org/10.1093/cid/cix1085.

21. Safdieh JE, Mead PA, Sepkowitz KA, et al. Bacterial and fungal meningitis in patients with cancer. Neurology 2008;70(12):943–7.
22. Lukes SA, Posner JB, Nielsen S, et al. Bacterial infections of the CNS in neutropenic patients. Neurology 1984;34(3):269–75.
23. Rosa RG, Goldani LZ. Cohort study of the impact of time to antibiotic administration on mortality in patients with febrile neutropenia. Antimicrob Agents Chemother 2014;58(7):3799–803.
24. Fiore AE, Fry A, Shay D, et al, Centers for Disease Control and Prevention (CDC). Antiviral agents for the treatment and chemoprophylaxis of influenza – recommendations of the Advisory Committee on Immunization Practices (ACIP). MMWR Recomm Rep 2011;60(1):1–24.
25. Casper C, Englund J, Boeckh M. How I treat influenza in patients with hematologic malignancies. Blood 2010;115(7):1331–42.
26. Gooskens J, Jonges M, Claas EC, et al. Prolonged influenza virus infection during lymphocytopenia and frequent detection of drug-resistant viruses. J Infect Dis 2009;199(10):1435–41.
27. Lee N, Chan PK, Choi KW, et al. Factors associated with early hospital discharge of adult influenza patients. Antivir Ther 2007;12(4):501–8.
28. Vu D, Peck AJ, Nichols WG, et al. Safety and tolerability of oseltamivir prophylaxis in hematopoietic stem cell transplant recipients: a retrospective case-control study. Clin Infect Dis 2007;45:187–93.
29. Monto AS, Fleming DM, Henry D, et al. Efficacy and safety of the neuraminidase inhibitor zanamivir in the treatment of influenza A and B virus infections. J Infect Dis 1999;180:254–61.
30. Nicholson KG, Aoki FY, Osterhaus AD, et al. Efficacy and safety of oseltamivir in treatment of acute influenza: a randomised controlled trial. Neuraminidase Inhibitor Flu Treatment Investigator Group. Lancet 2000;355:1845–50.
31. Kaiser L, Wat C, Mills T, et al. Impact of oseltamivir treatment on influenza-related lower respiratory tract complications and hospitalizations. Arch Intern Med 2003; 163:1667–72.
32. McGeer A, Green KA, Plevneshi A, et al. Antiviral therapy and outcomes of influenza requiring hospitalization in Ontario, Canada. Clin Infect Dis 2007;45: 1568–75.
33. Bautista E, Chotpitayasunondh T, Gao Z, et al. Clinical aspects of pandemic 2009 influenza A (H1N1) virus infection. N Engl J Med 2010;362:1708–19.
34. Rhodes A, Evans LE, Alhazzani W, et al. Surviving sepsis campaign: international guidelines for management of sepsis and septic shock: 2016. Crit Care Med 2017;45(3):486–552.
35. Klastersky J, Paesmans M, Rubenstein EB, et al. The Multinational Association for Supportive Care in Cancer risk index: a multinational scoring system for identifying low-risk febrile neutropenic cancer patients. J Clin Oncol 2000;18(16): 3038–51.
36. Uys A, Rapoport BL, Anderson R. Febrile neutropenia: a prospective study to validate the Multinational Association of Supportive Care of Cancer (MASCC) risk-index score. Support Care Cancer 2004;12(8):555–60.
37. Taj M, Nadeem M, Maqsood S, et al. Validation of MASCC Score for risk stratification in patients of hematological disorders with febrile neutropenia. Indian J Hematol Blood Transfus 2017;33(3):355–60.
38. Baskaran ND, Gan GG, Adeeba K. Applying the multinational association for supportive care in cancer risk scoring in predicting outcome of febrile neutropenia patients in a cohort of patients. Ann Hematol 2008;87(7):563–9.

39. Hui EP, Leung LK, Poon TC, et al. Prediction of outcome in cancer patients with febrile neutropenia: a prospective validation of the Multinational Association for Supportive Care in Cancer risk index in a Chinese population and comparison with the Talcott model and artificial neural network. Support Care Cancer 2011; 19(10):1625–35.
40. Klastersky J, Paesmans M. The multinational association for supportive care in cancer (MASCC) risk index score: 10 years of use for identifying low-risk febrile neutropenic cancer patients. Support Care Cancer 2013;21(5):1487–95.
41. Carmona-Bayonas A, Gómez J, González-Billalabeitia E, et al. Prognostic evaluation of febrile neutropenia in apparently stable adult cancer patients. Br J Cancer 2011;105(5):612–7.
42. Bitar RA. Utility of the Multinational Association for Supportive Care in Cancer (MASCC) risk index score as a criterion for nonadmission in febrile neutropenic patients with solid tumors. Perm J 2015;19(3):37–47.
43. Coyne CJ, Le V, Brennan JJ, et al. Application of the MASCC and CISNE risk-stratification scores to identify low-risk febrile neutropenic patients in the emergency department. Ann Emerg Med 2017;69(6):755–64.
44. Innes H, Lim SL, Hall A, et al. Management of febrile neutropenia in solid tumours and lymphomas using the Multinational Association for Supportive Care in Cancer (MASCC) risk index: feasibility and safety in routine clinical practice. Support Care Cancer 2008;16(5):485–91.
45. Cherif H, Johansson E, Björkholm M, et al. The feasibility of early hospital discharge with oral antimicrobial therapy in low risk patients with febrile neutropenia following chemotherapy for hematologic malignancies. Haematologica 2006; 91(2):215–22.
46. Klastersky J, Paesmans M, Georgala A, et al. Outpatient oral antibiotics for febrile neutropenic cancer patients using a score predictive for complications. J Clin Oncol 2006;24(25):4129–34.
47. Carmona-Bayonas A, Jiménez-Fonseca P, Virizuela Echaburu J, et al. Prediction of serious complications in patients with seemingly stable febrile neutropenia: validation of the clinical index of stable febrile neutropenia in a prospective cohort of patients from the FINITE study. J Clin Oncol 2015;33(5):465–71.
48. Marr KA. Infections in hematopoietic stem cell transplant recipients. In: Cohen J, Powderly WG, Opal SM, editors. Infectious diseases. 4th edition. China: Elsevier; 2017. p. 739–45.
49. Ramaprasad C, Pursell KJ. Infectious complications of stem cell transplantation. Cancer Treat Res 2014;161:351–70.
50. Tomblyn M, Chiller T, Einsele H, et al. Guidelines for preventing infectious complications among hematopoietic cell transplantation recipients: a global perspective. Biol Blood Marrow Transplant 2009;15(10):1143–238.
51. Caruana I, Diaconu I, Dotti G. From monoclonal antibodies to chimeric antigen receptors for the treatment of human malignancies. Semin Oncol 2014;41(5): 661–6.
52. Demlova R, Valík D, Obermannova R, et al. The safety of therapeutic monoclonal antibodies: implications for cancer therapy including immuno-checkpoint inhibitors. Physiol Res 2016;65(Suppl 4):S455–62.
53. Lee DW, Gardner R, Porter DL, et al. Current concepts in the diagnosis and management of cytokine release syndrome. Blood 2014;124(2):188–95.
54. Frey NV, Porter DL. Cytokine release syndrome with novel therapeutics for acute lymphoblastic leukemia. Hematology Am Soc Hematol Educ Program 2016;2016: 567–72.

55. Neelapu SS, Tummala S, Kebriaei P, et al. Chimeric antigen receptor T-cell therapy - assessment and management of toxicities. Nat Rev Clin Oncol 2017. https://doi.org/10.1038/nrclinonc.2017.148.
56. Brudno JN, Kochenderfer JN. Toxicities of chimeric antigen receptor T cells: recognition and management. Blood 2016;127(26):3321–30.
57. Bonifant CL, Jackson HJ, Brentjens RJ, et al. Toxicity and management in CAR T-cell therapy. Mol Ther Oncolytics 2016;3:16011.

Rapid Fire: Tumor Lysis Syndrome

Sarah B. Dubbs, MD

KEYWORDS

- Tumor lysis syndrome • Uric acid • Rasburicase • Metabolic emergency • Cancer
- Emergency

KEY POINTS

- Tumor lysis syndrome (TLS) is a life-threatening metabolic complication of cancer.
- TLS is characterized by a constellation of metabolic derangements stemming from the release of intracellular products: hyperkalemia, hyperuricemia, hyperphosphatemia, and hypocalcemia.
- These metabolic derangements lead to end-organ damage, including renal failure, dysrhythmias, and neurologic involvement.
- Management is centered on hydration, reduction of uric acid, and treatment of electrolyte abnormalities.

CASE

Pertinent history: A 47-year-old woman with no significant medical history presents for evaluation of progressive fatigue, generalized weakness, nausea, and diffuse muscle cramps for 2 weeks. She denies chest pain or diaphoresis but does say that she now has shortness of breath with minimal exertion. She has not had cough, fevers, abdominal pain, or diarrhea.

Past medical history: no chronic medical problems

Surgical history: cesarean delivery, cholecystectomy

Medications: none

Family history: hypertension in mother and father; no known coronary disease of venous thromboembolism history in family

Social history: no tobacco or illicit drug use; social alcohol use

Pertinent physical examination: Temperature: 37.3; blood pressure: 105/56; heart rate: 112; Respiratory Rate = 21; oxygen saturation as measured by pulse oximetry: 99% on room air

General: alert, ill appearing, oriented × 3

Disclosure Statement: The author has no relationship with a commercial company that has a direct financial interest in the subject matter or materials discussed in the article or with a company making a competing product.

Department of Emergency Medicine, University of Maryland School of Medicine, 110 South Paca Street, 6th Floor, Suite 200, Baltimore, MD 21201, USA

E-mail address: sdubbs@som.umaryland.edu

Emerg Med Clin N Am 36 (2018) 517–525
https://doi.org/10.1016/j.emc.2018.04.003
0733-8627/18/© 2018 Elsevier Inc. All rights reserved.

Head/Eyes/Ears/Nose/Throat: PERRL, mucous membranes dry, conjunctivae pale
Neck: full range of motion (ROM), neck veins flat
Cardiovascular: regular rhythm, tachycardic, no murmurs/rubs/gallops, distal pulses equal bilaterally
Pulmonary: rate increased but speaks in full sentences; lungs clear with no wheezes, rales, or rhonchi
Abdominal: soft, nontender, nondistended, normal bowel sounds
Neurologic: 5/5 strength and normal sensation throughout
Musculoskeletal: normal pulses throughout, full ROM of all extremities, no significant peripheral edema
Skin: petechial rash scattered on lower extremities

Diagnostic testing: A cardiac workup is initiated.

WBC	58.3 K/mcL
Hgb	9.2 g/dL
Hct	25.4%
Plt	19 K/mcL
ANC	0.9 K/mcL
Na	132 mmol/L
Potassium	7.1 mmol/L
Cl	101 mmol/L
CO_2	21 mmol/L
Glucose	99 mg/dL
BUN	21 mg/dL
Creatinine	2.3 mg/dL
Calcium	5.1 mg/dL
Troponin	<0.02 ng/mL

Abbreviations: ANC, absolute neutrophil count; BUN, serum urea nitrogen; Cl, chloride; CO_2, carbon dioxide; Hct, hematocrit; Hgb, hemoglobin; Plt, platelet; WBC, white blood cell.

Electrocardiogram (EKG): sinus tachycardia; normal axis and intervals; no ST elevation or depression; T waves peaked and pointed
Chest radiograph: normal

Clinical course: Based on the patient's initial presentation, a cardiac workup was initiated with EKG, laboratory tests, and chest radiograph. The EKG was obtained first and revealed T-wave changes concerning for hyperkalemia. Intravenous calcium was ordered and was administered, as the remainder of the laboratory tests resulted.

The patient was found to have a marked leukocytosis, anemia, and thrombocytopenia, raising suspicion for acute leukemia. An automated differential found her to have profound neutropenia as well. The suspected hyperkalemia was confirmed, and she was also found to have renal failure and low calcium. Additional treatment was ordered for the hyperkalemia. Her troponin was normal, and the chest film did not show signs of overt fluid overload. Additional laboratory studies were ordered to further investigate the patient's metabolic abnormalities.

LEARNING POINTS
Introduction and Background

- Tumor lysis syndrome (TLS) is a life-threatening metabolic complication of cancer, characterized by life-threatening hyperkalemia, hyperuricemia, hyperphosphatemia, and hypocalcemia as a result of massive lysis of cells.
- Morbidity worldwide seems to be decreasing because of improved prophylaxis and vigilance to detect the complication; however, prompt diagnosis and treatment by emergency physicians is essential to improved outcomes in these patients.

Physiology/Pathophysiology

1. TLS is characterized by a constellation of metabolic derangements stemming from the release of intracellular products.
2. Although it can occur spontaneously in hematologic malignancies or highly proliferative solid tumors (autolysis), TLS most often occurs within a few hours to days after administration of cytotoxic chemotherapy.[1]
   - Types of cancers most susceptible to developing TLS with chemotherapy:
     a. Rapidly growing, chemosensitive myelo-lymphoproliferative cancers with high white blood cell counts, such as acute leukemias
     b. Cancers with large, bulky adenopathy, such as high-grade non-Hodgkin lymphomas
   - TLS has also been reported in patients who have received ionizing radiation, embolization, radiofrequency ablation, monoclonal antibody therapy, glucocorticoids, interferon, and hematopoietic stem cell transplantation.[2]
3. Cell lysis results in the release of potassium, nucleic acids (which metabolize to uric acid), phosphorus, and other metabolites into the bloodstream, leading to systemic end-organ effects. **Fig. 1** summarizes the major features of TLS.
   - *Hyperkalemia* poses the most immediate danger in TLS, as it can cause life-threatening cardiac dysrhythmia and sudden death.
   - Purine nucleic acids are catabolized first to hypoxanthine. Xanthine oxidase catabolizes the hypoxanthine to xanthine and then to *uric acid*. Uric acid is not excreted well by the kidneys. Humans, in fact, lack the enzyme that further breaks uric acid down into the much more soluble allantoin. This enzyme is called uricase. In TLS, the overwhelming amount of uric acid that cannot be excreted leads to uric acid crystal precipitation and nephropathy (**Fig. 2**).
   - *Phosphorus* binds extracellular calcium and precipitates into calcium phosphate crystals (see **Fig. 2**). The binding of calcium depletes the calcium supply, causing *hypocalcemia*.
     a. Severe hypocalcemia may cause paresthesias, muscle cramps, tetany, seizures, or cardiac dysrhythmias.
     b. Calcium phosphate crystals deposit in the renal tubules causing nephropathy.
   - Intravascular volume depletion and acute renal failure may also cause lactic acidosis.
   - These metabolic derangements often manifest with systemic symptoms, such as fatigue, nausea/vomiting, generalized weakness, and altered mental status.

Making the Diagnosis

1. Emergency physicians must be vigilant in the detection of TLS in patients with established cancers, as well as those without prior oncologic diagnosis, but who are found to have the hallmark metabolic derangements of the syndrome.
2. The presentation of TLS ranges from asymptomatic laboratory abnormalities to severe end-organ/multiorgan failure to death.

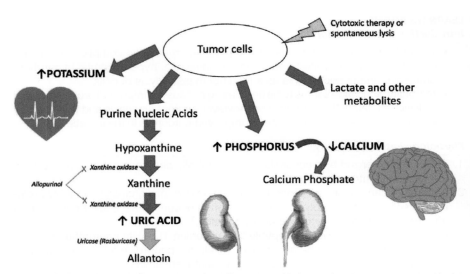

Fig. 1. Pathophysiology of TLS. Tumor lysis (by cytotoxic chemotherapy, spontaneous lysis, or other cause) releases potassium, nucleic acids (which are catabolized to uric acid), and phosphorus, which precipitates with calcium, lactate, and other metabolites, causing life-threatening end-organ damage. Also shown is the mechanism of action of allopurinol, which lowers uric acid production by inhibiting the xanthine oxidase enzyme, and the mechanism of action of rasburicase, which converts uric acid to the much more soluble allantoin.

3. Patients suspected of having TLS should undergo diagnostic testing that includes, at minimum, the following:
   - Basic metabolic panel
   - Calcium
   - Phosphorus
   - Uric acid
   - Lactate
   - Urinalysis

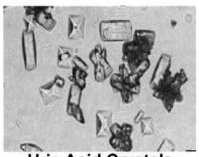

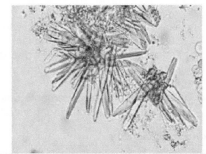

Uric Acid Crystals   Calcium Phosphate Crystals

Fig. 2. Uric acid and calcium phosphate crystals on urine microscopy. (*Courtesy of* Colin. Kaide, MD, Wexner Medical Center at The Ohio State University Columbus, Ohio, USA; with permission.)

- EKG
- Other diagnostics pertinent to the presenting symptoms and differential diagnosis
4. **Table 1** summarizes the Cairo and Bishop classification system for TLS. TLS is classified into laboratory and clinical TLS[1]:
   - Laboratory TLS: abnormality in 2 or more of the following, occurring within 3 days prior or 7 days after chemotherapy:
     a. Potassium $\geq$6 mEq/L or 25% increase from baseline
     b. Uric acid $\geq$8 mg/dL or 25% increase from baseline
     c. Phosphate $\geq$4.5 mg/dL or 25% increase from baseline
     d. Calcium $\leq$7 mg/dL or 25% decrease from baseline
   - Clinical TLS: laboratory TLS plus 1 or more of the following:
     a. Creatinine $\geq$1.5$\times$ upper limit of normal (ULN)
     b. Cardiac dysrhythmia
     c. Seizure
5. Cairo and Bishop also developed a severity grading system for TLS, summarized in **Tables 2** and **3**. The grading ranges from grade 0 (creatinine $\geq$1.5 or greater $\times$ ULN and no cardiac arrhythmia or seizure) to grade 5 (death).
6. As noted previously, the workup should be guided by patients' presenting symptoms, as they may have multiple emergent issues in addition to TLS.

Treating Patients

1. Patients undergoing cancer treatment are monitored closely by their oncologists with routine surveillance laboratory tests. Those at higher risk (based on tumor burden, risk of cell lysis, organ function and preexisting conditions) undergo preventative measures, such as intravenous hydration, allopurinol, and oral phosphate binders, before chemotherapy.[3]
2. Once laboratory or clinical TLS has been identified, treatment is guided by the severity of the laboratory derangements and clinical manifestations. Most major cancer centers have developed local treatment guidelines for TLS. Reviewed here are the general tenants of TLS treatment.
   - Hydration
     a. Aggressive hydration is one of the most important interventions and should begin immediately[2]; however, it should be undertaken cautiously in patients with significant renal failure, oliguria, or congestive heart failure.
     b. The goal of hydration is to improve renal perfusion and glomerular filtration rate, aiming for urine output of at least 2 mL/kg/h.[3]
     c. Loop diuretics may also be used to augment urine output in those who are not volume depleted.

Table 1	
Cairo and Bishop classification system for tumor lysis syndrome	
Laboratory TLS	**Clinical TLS**
Abnormality in $\geq$2 of the following, occurring within 3 d prior or 7 d after chemotherapy:	*Laboratory TLS* plus $\geq$1 of the following:
• *Potassium* $\geq$6 mEq/L or 25% increase from baseline	• *Creatinine* $\geq$1.5$\times$ ULN
• *Uric acid* $\geq$8 mg/dL or 25% increase from baseline	• Cardiac dysrhythmia
• *Phosphate* $\geq$4.5 mg/dL or 25% increase from baseline	• Seizure
• *Calcium* $\leq$7 mg/dL or 25% decrease from baseline	

Abbreviation: ULN, upper limit of normal.

Adapted from Cairo MS, Bishop M. Tumor lysis syndrome: new therapeutic strategies and classification. Br J Haematol 2004;127(1):3–11; with permission.

Table 2
Cairo-Bishop grading classification of tumor lysis syndrome

	Grade 0[a]	Grade I	Grade II	Grade III	Grade IV	Grade V
LTLS	−	+	+	+	+	+
Creatinine[b,c]	≤1.5 × ULN	1.5 × ULN	>1.5–3 0 × ULN	>3.0–6.0 × ULN	>6.0 ULN	Death[d]
Cardiac arrhythmia[c]	None	Intervention not indicated	Nonurgent medical intervention indicated	Symptomatic and incompletely controlled medically or controlled with device (eg, defibrillator)	Life-threatening (eg, arrhythmia associated with CHF, hypotension, syncope, shock)	Death[d]
Seizure[c]	None	—	One brief generalized seizure; seizures well controlled by anticonvulsant or infrequent focal motor seizures not interfering with ADLs	Seizure in which consciousness is altered; poorly controlled seizure disorder; with breakthrough generalized seizures despite medical intervention	Seizure of any kind that is prolonged, repetitive, or difficult to control (eg, status epilepticus, intractable epilepsy)	Death[d]

Clinical TLS (CTLS) requires one or more clinical manifestations along with criteria for laboratory TLS. Maximal CTLS manifestation (renal, cardiac, neuro) defines the grade.

Abbreviations: ADLs, activities of daily living; CHF, congestive heart failure; LTLS, laboratory TLS.

[a] No laboratory TLS.

[b] Creatinine levels: Patients will be considered to have elevated creatinine if their serum creatinine is 1.5 times greater than the institutional ULN less than the age/sex-defined ULN. If not specified by an institution, age/sex ULN creatinine may be defined as follows: greater than 1 year to less than 12 years of age, both male and female, 61.6 μmol/L; 12 years to less than 16 years of age, both male and female, 88 μmol/L; 16 years of age or older, female, 105.6 μmol/L; 16 years of age or older, male 114.4 μmol/L.

[c] Not directly or probably attributable to a therapeutic agent (eg, increase in creatinine after amphotericin administration).

[d] Attributive probably or definitely to clinical TLS.

From Cairo MS, Bishop M. Tumor lysis syndrome: new therapeutic strategies and classification. Br J Haematol 2004;127(1):6; with permission.

Table 3
Clinical features of the metabolic abnormalities found in tumor lysis syndrome

Abnormality	Clinical Features
Hyperkalemia	• EKG changes and dysrhythmia • Myalgias, weakness, paresthesias • Nausea, vomiting, diarrhea
Hyperuricemia	• Renal failure
Hyperphosphatemia	• Renal failure • Secondary hypocalcemia
Hypocalcemia	• Muscle spasm, tetany, paresthesias • Altered mental status • Seizure

- Reduce uric acid
  a. Allopurinol
     i. Allopurinol is an analogue of hypoxanthine and lowers uric acid by inhibiting xanthine oxidase, therefore, inhibiting the conversion of hypoxanthine to xanthine to uric acid (see **Fig. 1**). Allopurinol's active metabolite also inhibits xanthine oxidase.
     ii. Allopurinol only inhibits the synthesis of uric acid. It does not have an effect on preexisting uric acid, making it essentially ineffective on uric acid levels in the first 48 to 72 hours of treatment.[2]
  b. Rasburicase
     i. Rasburicase is a recombinant urate oxidase (uricase). Uricase is the enzyme that converts uric acid into the more urine soluble allantoin (see **Fig. 1**).
     ii. Because uric acid is degraded by this medication, the levels are immediately reduced after administration.
  c. Alkalinization
     i. Urine alkalinization for treatment of hyperuricemia in TLS is no longer recommended.
     ii. Alkalinization of urine theoretically promotes uric acid excretion, as it increases its solubility; however, it increases precipitation of calcium phosphate at the same time, worsening renal damage and hypocalcemia.
- Treat electrolyte abnormalities
  a. Hyperkalemia
     i. Cardiac dysrhythmias and sudden death from hyperkalemia are the most immediate life-threating results from TLS. Fortunately, they are also conditions with which emergency physicians are very comfortable and treat routinely.
     ii. Signs of hyperkalemia can be detected early with EKG. Peaked T waves, widened QRS, and other EKG signs of severe hyperkalemia may prompt empirical treatment before laboratory results have returned.
     iii. Hyperkalemia in TLS should be approached in the same fashion as hyperkalemia due to any other cause with calcium to stabilize the myocardium, insulin/hypertonic dextrose, albuterol, sodium bicarbonate, loops diuretics, and/or dialysis. In addition to stabilizing the myocardium, supplementing calcium will also mitigate TLS-related hypocalcemia (which will also correct with treatment of hyperphosphatemia). Note that excess calcium could, however, lead to increased calcium phosphate precipitation.
  b. Hyperphosphatemia and hypocalcemia
     i. Moderate hyperphosphatemia is generally treated with hydration, restriction of phosphorus intake, and oral phosphate binders.

    ii. Severe hyperphosphatemia may require hemodialysis. Insulin and hypertonic dextrose may also be used to acutely shift severe hyperphosphatemia.

    iii. Treating hyperphosphatemia will improve hypocalcemia secondarily. If patients are symptomatic with muscular spasm, tetany, paresthesia, altered mental status, or seizures, intravenous calcium can be administered slowly as not to encourage precipitation with phosphorus.

3. Patients undergoing treatment of TLS should have frequent laboratory monitoring every 4 to 6 hours and remain in a cardiac-monitored setting. Unless asymptomatic, most will require a higher level of care in an intermediate care unit or intensive care unit.

4. Always discuss and coordinate care with the appropriate consultants, namely, oncology, nephrology, and critical care.

CASE CONCLUSION

The additional laboratory test results that were ordered included a uric acid level, phosphorus level, lactate level, and urinalysis, on the suspicion of TLS caused by the patient's hematologic malignancy. The uric acid, phosphorus, and lactate levels were elevated; the urinalysis showed ketones and crystals. Aggressive intravenous fluid hydration was initiated with a goal urine output of 2 mL/kg/h, and rasburicase was given in consultation with oncology. Nephrology was also consulted and on standby in case the patient required hemodialysis. She was admitted, given allopurinol and oral phosphate binders, more hydration, and underwent a bone marrow biopsy confirming the diagnosis of acute lymphocytic leukemia. Once her TLS improved, she was started on induction chemotherapy.

DISCUSSION

With the incidence of cancer continuing to grow, emergency physicians are faced with the responsibility of diagnosing and treating all types of oncologic emergencies. TLS continues to carry high morbidity, though early detection and treatment can be very effective in limiting its progression. The key to swift diagnosis in the emergency department is carrying a high clinical suspicion in high-risk patients as well as recognizing the pattern of TLS findings in those who are presenting with their cardinal presentation of cancer (such as the woman in the featured case). Prompt recognition, treatment, and coordination of care will most certainly pay dividends in days and quality of life for the patients at hand.

Pattern recognition

TLS

- Common in acute leukemias and lymphomas or other highly proliferative solid tumors, often within several days of chemotherapy
- Hyperkalemia
- Hyperuricemia
- Hyperphosphatemia/hypocalcemia
- Renal failure
- Urine crystals
- Treatment: hydrate, treat electrolytes, decrease uric acid

REFERENCES

1. Cairo MS, Bishop M. Tumor lysis syndrome: new therapeutic strategies and classification. Br J Haematol 2004;127(1):3–11.
2. Fojo AT. Metabolic emergencies. In: Devita VT Jr, Lawrence TS, Rosenberg SA, editors. Cancer principles and practice of oncology. 10th edition. Philadelphia: Wolters Kluwer Health; 2015. p. 1822–31.
3. Howard SC, Jones DP, Pui C-H. The tumor lysis syndrome. N Engl J Med 2011;364: 1844–54.

Pediatric Oncologic Emergencies

Kathleen Stephanos, MD[a,b,*], Lindsey Picard, MD[b]

KEYWORDS

- Pediatric oncology • Tumor lysis syndrome • Typhlitis
- Pediatric cancer emergencies

KEY POINTS

- Pediatric cancer often presents as vague complaints, many times with more common medical issues on the differential diagnosis.
- Parents and children should be informed of the diagnosis in an age-appropriate and timely fashion.
- Although many treatment management strategies for chemotherapy complications remain the same throughout all age groups, there are pediatric-specific considerations when evaluating these patients.

CASE 1

A 10-year-old boy presents with several weeks of generalized symptoms. He reports malaise, increased sleeping, easy fatigability, and some night sweats. His parents have noted that he appears more pale than usual. They initially thought he had a viral illness but over time he continued to have symptoms and was seen by his primary care doctor who reported some slight anemia on bloodwork. He has gradually developed some atraumatic lower back pain.

social history: lives with mother, father, and an older sister.

past medical history: none.

Medications: none.

Vital signs: blood pressure 96 over 60, pulse 115, temperature 37.2°, respiratory rate 18, pulse oximetry 97%.

General: alert and oriented x3, tired appearing, baggy clothes.

Eyes: conjunctivae normal; pupils are equal, round, and reactive to light.

Neck: supple, no jugular venous distension.

Disclosure Statement: No financial disclosures for either author.
[a] Department of Pediatrics, University of Rochester, 601 Elmwood Avenue Box 655, Rochester, NY 14642, USA; [b] Department of Emergency Medicine, University of Rochester, 601 Elmwood Avenue Box 655, Rochester, NY 14642, USA
* Corresponding author. 601 Elmwood Avenue Box 655, Rochester, NY 14642.
E-mail address: Kathleen_stephanos@urmc.rochester.edu

Emerg Med Clin N Am 36 (2018) 527–535
https://doi.org/10.1016/j.emc.2018.04.007
0733-8627/18/© 2018 Elsevier Inc. All rights reserved.
emed.theclinics.com

Cardiovascular: heart with regular rate and rhythm, normal heart sounds, intact distal pulses throughout. No gallop, no rub.

Pulmonary or chest: no respiratory distress, no wheezes, no tenderness.

Abdomen: scaphoid upper abdomen, which is soft and nontender. Lower abdomen firm with palpable mass to the umbilicus. Palpation produces a need to urinate but no tenderness.

Neurological assessment: cranial nerves intact, strength intact throughout, sensation intact throughout.

Extremities: no edema, no tenderness, no deformities.

Skin: areas of bruising from prior minor injuries, no petechiae.

Diagnostic tests	
White Blood Cell Count	20.9×10^9/L
Hemoglobin	7.5 g/dL
Hematocrit	23%
Platelet level	64×10^9/L
Sodium	138 mEq/L
Potassium	5.0 mEq/L
Chloride	101 mEq/L
Creatinine	1.12 mEq/L
Carbon dioxide	21 mEq/L
Blood urea nitrogen	10 mEq/L
Phosphate	4.2 mEq/L
Calcium	6.9 mEq/L

GENERAL INTRODUCTORY OR BACKGROUND

Pediatric cancers are the leading cause of death due to disease in children in developed countries, second only to injuries in pediatrics deaths overall.[1] The most common forms are leukemia, central nervous system (CNS) tumors, lymphoma, soft tissue, renal or pelvic (neuroblastoma), and bone tumors.[2] It is important to consider other congenital medical history because some syndromes have higher cancer associations.[3]

PATHOPHYSIOLOGY

1. Many pediatric cancers result in anemia. In leukemia this is a direct result of bone marrow infiltration. By contrast, in many of the other forms, inflammatory cytokines result in a decrease in blood cell production. Although large masses can have necrosis with bleeding into the tumor, resulting in hemorrhagic blood loss, anemia tends to be normocytic normochromic.[4]
2. Tumor lysis can be a direct result of a tumor involuting due to high tumor burden or due to initial treatment. Usually, the latter occurs while a patient is admitted. Tumor lysis syndrome occurs owing to increased cellular turnover and death, resulting in intracellular content release into the blood, which in turn causes the release or intracellular DNA and electrolytes. This can cause cardiac instability and arrhythmias, as well as renal failure. Less commonly, this may cause seizure due to electrolyte disturbances. Children with a baseline renal dysfunction are at higher risk for tumor lysis syndrome.[5]

3. Hyperleukocytosis is defined as a white blood cell count of greater than 100,000 and can result in leukostasis, predominantly causing pulmonary or CNS symptoms.[4]
4. Altered mental status can result from tumor burden within the CNS, which, in extreme cases, can result in herniation. In pediatrics this is often due to primary brain masses and CNS fluid infiltration by leukemia. Secondary metastases as a cause are rarer in children, whereas they are relatively common in adults. Additionally, hyperviscosity as a result of leukemia can also increase risk of stroke, resulting in an altered mental status and seizures.
5. Respiratory distress can be the result of mass lesions, most commonly associated with lymphoma, and have a 60% risk of airway compromise.[6]
6. Superior vena cava syndrome (SVCS) occurs by external compression and prevention of the blood flow by a tumor or blood clot. This occurs owing to the thin-walled nature of the superior vena cava, which makes it easily compressible.[7]
7. Bowel obstruction or intussusception can occur due to tumor burden compressing the bowel or acting as a lead point for intussusception. Tumor must be considered in children older than 2 to 3 years of age presenting with intussusception, and in all children with unexplained bowel obstruction.[4]
8. Pathologic fractures can occur due to primary bone tumors.[4]

MAKING THE DIAGNOSIS

1. History
   - Many pediatric patients with cancer present with vague symptoms such as fatigue, headaches, unexplained long bone pain, fevers, weight loss, pallor, or anemia (if laboratory samples are drawn).[8]
2. Examination findings
   - Generalized pallor is common in many forms of pediatrics cancers owing to anemia.[3]
   - Mediastinal mass should be considered in a patient with new wheezing symptoms, particularly in children who are school age, and must be addressed before steroid administration.[6]
   - Altered mental status, focal neurologic deficits, and seizures without return to baseline should cause concern for an intracranial pathologic condition.[8]
   - The brachial vein remaining full with right arm lift is an indication of SVCS. Facial swelling, arm swelling, full jugular veins, cyanosis, or plethora are also common findings of this diagnosis.[7]
   - Intermittent abdominal pain, vomiting, and decreased stool output or bloody stools may indicate an intraabdominal pathologic condition.[3]
   - Bruising, bleeding, and petechiae can suggest thrombocytopenia.[4]
   - Increased blood pressure should prompt the provider to consider neuroblastoma or a renal pathologic condition.[3]
   - Cardiac arrhythmia and arrest can occur owing to tumor lysis.[9]
3. Laboratory findings
   - Nonspecific laboratory findings occur in pediatric cancers overall.
   - Anemia and thrombocytopenia can occur with all forms.
   - Tumor lysis laboratory findings include hyperkalemia, hyperphosphatemia, hypocalcemia, elevated lactate dehydrogenase, increased uric acid, and renal failure.[5]
4. Imaging
   - Often, imaging is obtained at the discretion of pediatric hematology or oncology. These providers should be consulted for nonemergent studies to help obtain complete evaluations and avoid unnecessary radiation exposure in children.

- Chest radiograph may show a mediastinal mass.
- Head computed tomography is indicated in cases of altered mental status and with seizures without return to baseline.
- Abdominal ultrasound can be used as initial imaging for mass lesions or concern for intussusception.
- Free air abdominal series can be obtained for cases of concern for obstruction.
- Imaging of bones may reveal a mass or pathologic fracture.

TREATING THE PATIENT

1. Unlike adult patients, most new cancer diagnoses in children warrant an admission.
2. New cancer diagnoses are particularly challenging within the pediatric population. A discussion with the parents should occur separate from the child, with an assessment of how they think the child should be informed. It is important that the child be notified in age-appropriate terminology shortly thereafter. There is evidence that delayed patient information results in patient anxiety and distrust in both the family and medical providers in the future and can have long-term implications.[10]
3. Tumor lysis is primarily managed with intravenous fluids. Allopurinol and rasburicase can be added to the regimen in patients with complications of tumor lysis or in those presenting in severe forms (renal failure or altered mental status). These medications are usually added at the discretion of the oncologist. Allopurinol decreases the production of uric acid, and rasburicase increases uric acid metabolism. The goals are to prevent arrhythmia, renal failure, altered mental status, and (ultimately) multiorgan failure.[5]
4. Hyperleukocytosis should be managed with high-volume fluids and may require leukapheresis or immediate initiation of chemotherapy at the direction of oncology. With these patients, blood transfusion may worsen symptoms; therefore, if the patient is stable, blood transfusion should be withheld.[8]
5. Signs of increased intracranial pressure should be managed similarly to other patients with these symptoms. Placing the head of the bed upright, hyperventilation (a temporizing measure for up to 30 minutes), and hypertonic saline may be used for signs of impending herniation.[4]
6. Seizures can be managed with typical antiepileptics, though electrolyte management may be a necessary component of management.[4]
7. Respiratory compromise may require intubation. Mediastinal masses may require the bed to be upright to avoid compression. It is essential to avoid steroids in new childhood wheezing until a mass is reasonably excluded because this can initiate some treatment and limit the efficacy of future biopsy.[6]
8. Management of SVCS may require stenting or anticoagulation, depending on the cause. The head of bed should be kept upright to improve blood return. These patients require an intensive care unit level of care.[7]
9. Bowel obstructions are managed per typical guidelines and may respond to bowel rest.

CASE SUMMARY

Imaging confirmed a mass present within the lower pelvis, resulting in ureteral obstruction and bilateral hydronephrosis. The patient was admitted to the pediatric oncology service for biopsy and evaluation. Biopsy results confirmed Burkitt lymphoma. Ureteral stents were placed and he was started on chemotherapy.

CASE DISCUSSION

There are multiple red flags present in this case that should always prompt further evaluation in pediatric patients. Cancers should be suspected in those presenting with prolonged fevers, unexplained fatigue, unexplained weight loss, atraumatic back pain, or new anemia. Unlike adults in whom specifically unexplained weight loss is a concern, cases of growing children with any weight loss should raise some red flags. Tumors should also be considered in children presenting with headaches. Although many of these symptoms have other explanations in adult patients, children rarely have this constellation of symptoms and are generally more resilient and able to ignore minor injuries, strains, and sprains that will cause adults to seek care.

Pattern recognition

- Weight loss in a growing child
- Normocytic, normochromic anemia
- Electrolyte derangements, specifically
  - Hyperkalemia
  - Hyperphosphatemia
  - Hyperuricemia
  - Hypocalcemia
  - Elevated LDH
- Unexplained bruising or bleeding
- Persistent, unexplained pain, particularly in back or long bones
- New onset wheezing
- Mental status changes.

CASE 2

A 10-year-old boy undergoing treatment for Burkitt lymphoma presents with fever, nausea, mouth pain, and vague abdominal discomfort. He recently completed induction chemotherapy and was neutropenic at his last check the day before presentation. He reports nonspecific abdominal discomfort associated with a fever at home to 100.7°. He has no known sick contacts and has experienced no complications so far with treatment. His appetite has been decreased and he has loose nonbloody stools since starting treatment.

SH: he lives with mother, father, and an older sister.

PMH: Burkitt lymphoma requiring prior red blood cell and platelet transfusions and with tumor lysis on initiation of chemotherapy.

Medications: cyclophosphamide, doxorubicin, methotrexate, vincristine.

Vital signs: blood pressure 86 over 60, pulse 120, temperature 39.2°, RR 25, SpO2 93%.

General: alert and oriented x3, tired appearing.

Head, ear, eye, nose, throat (HEENT): conjunctivae normal; pupils are equal, round, and reactive to light; lips dry, red mucous membranes.

Neck: supple, no JVD.

Cardiovascular: heart with regular rate and rhythm, normal heart sounds, intact distal pulses throughout. No gallop, no rub.

Pulmonary or chest: no respiratory distress, no wheezes, no tenderness.

Abdomen: soft, diffusely tender, no focal peritonitis, no palpable masses.

Neurological assessment: cranial nerves intact, strength intact throughout, sensation intact throughout.

Extremities: no edema, no tenderness, no deformities.

Skin: areas of bruising from prior minor injuries, no petechiae.

Diagnostic testing	
White Blood Cell Count	0.2×10^9/L
Neutrophils	0.2×10^9/L
Hemoglobin	9 g/dL
Hematocrit	26%
Platelet level	76×10^9/L
Sodium	134 mEq/L
Potassium	4.7 mEq/L
Chloride	100 mEq/L
Creatinine	0.90 mEq/L
Carbon dioxide	19 mEq/L
Blood urea nitrogen	20 mEq/L

GENERAL INTRODUCTORY OR BACKGROUND

Complications of cancer treatment are very common and are often an expected occurrence during treatment. As survival and recognition of pediatric cancers and treatments improve, the number of patients who are home on therapy has increased, resulting in an increase in emergency presentations that may have previously been only seen while in the hospital. Although some complications are direct known side effects of treatment, others are complications related to those side effects.[8]

PATHOPHYSIOLOGY

1. Blood dyscrasias are extremely common and include anemia, neutropenia, and thrombocytopenia. Goals for hemoglobin or hematocrit and platelet levels can depend on the patient and therapeutic agent. These are generally caused by bone marrow suppression from chemotherapeutic agents.[8]
2. Patients may have neutropenia due to therapy that predisposed them to a variety of viral, bacterial, and fungal infections. This can result in a rapid and severe response when a patient with neutropenia presents with a fever.[11]
3. Chemotherapeutic agent use can weaken the intraabdominal lumen, predisposing patients to perforation.[12]
4. Coagulopathy due to medications can result in hemorrhages or clots.[4]
5. Typhlitis, also known as neutropenic enterocolitis, is a predominantly pediatric cancer complication that occurs owing to bacterial or fungal invasion of the bowel wall in severely neutropenic patients. Its true pathophysiology is unclear but it occurs mainly in leukemia patients with neutrophil counts less than 500.[12]
6. There is generally delayed presentation of intraabdominal catastrophe, including appendicitis, due to immunosuppression.[12]
7. Mucositis occurs owing to chemotherapeutics causing breakdown of the mucosal tissues and can occur anywhere within the gastrointestinal tract, resulting in pain, risk of infection, bleeding, and dehydration.[13,14]

8. Multiple medications have the side effect of hypercoagulability, which can result in stroke, SVCS, or other ischemic disease.[8]
9. Iron overload is a complication of multiple transfusions.[8]

MAKING THE DIAGNOSIS

1. History
   - Neutropenic patients are at high risk and may have few to no presenting symptoms other than vague complaints such as vomiting, abdominal pain (without peritonitis), or fever.[11]
   - It is important to know the last chemotherapy treatment date, medications, prior complications, and timing of symptoms in relation to a treatment.[4]
2. Examination findings
   - Neutropenic patients can appear well or only mildly ill with severe life-threatening infections.[11]
   - Nothing should enter an orifice in evaluation of a neutropenic patient. This includes no rectal examination and no urinary catheterizations.[11]
   - Abdominal pain can be a sign of many highly concerning intraabdominal processes such as thrombosis, typhlitis, or appendicitis.[4]
   - Fever should prompt immediate consideration of neutropenic fever and a rapid workup with early initiation of antibiotics.
3. Laboratory findings
   - Calculate the absolute neutrophil count.

Absolute neutrophil count (ANC) calculation, in which WBC is white blood cell.

ANC = (% neutrophils + % bands) × WBC count (cells/μL)

Example: WBC = 2000 (cells/μL) + neutrophils = 10% and bands = 2%

Then ANC = 12% × 2000 (cells/μL) = 240 (cells/μL)

   - Laboratory findings are generally specific to the diagnosis and may be normal but a complete blood count is generally indicated in all patients.

4. Imaging
   - The choice of imaging type depends on presentation.
   - An abdominal radiograph free air series may show intestinal pneumatosis in typhlitis[12] but does not rule it out.
   - Computed tomography should be considered in any patient with peritonitis owing to the high risk of a pathologic condition; it should not be delayed by obtaining a less specific imaging such as ultrasound.

TREATMENT

1. Blood dyscrasias can be treated to meet the goals of care as defined by the treating oncologist. When transfusing, irradiated blood should be used. Irradiated blood prevents transfusion-associated graft-versus-host disease. Additionally, patients should be tested for cytomegalovirus (CMV) at initiation of treatment. Many pediatric patients are negative, unlike adults, and exposure during treatment can be fatal, so CMV negative blood should be used.[4]
2. Neutropenic fever should prompt antibiotics, monotherapy with ampicillin-sulbactam or cefepime, in well-appearing patients and those with no known resistance. Vancomycin should be added for ill-appearing patients and those with

known drug-resistance profiles that indicate its use. It should be considered (though not automatically added) for patients with ports or other tubing. Pediatric oncology should participate in discussions early in care to ensure appropriate patient-directed care.[11]

3. Intraabdominal processes should prompt early surgical consultation and the use of broad-spectrum antibiotics.[12] Surgical care should be carefully coordinated with oncology.
4. Mucositis can be managed by symptomatic pain control and fluids for signs of dehydration. This may require admission if significant symptoms prevent appropriate oral hydration.[13]
5. Thrombotic events may require initiation of anticoagulation but, again, this should be at the discretion of oncology.[4]

CASE SUMMARY

The patient was admitted and treated for neutropenic fever and dehydration with antibiotics and intravenous fluids. Abdominal pain improved with hydration. No source was identified in work-up; therefore, the illness was presumed to be viral in nature.

CASE DISCUSSION

This patient, like many oncology patients, presented with vague symptoms. After initiation of treatment, patients may present owing to either medication side effects or illnesses that can rapidly progress. Pediatric patients are more prone to dehydration, and they may be more limited in their willingness or ability to hydrate. Pediatric patients do develop fever more readily in response to viral processes than adults, making assessment for a viral cause of their symptoms very important, in addition to maintaining a high suspicion for bacterial infections and other complications.

Pattern recognition

- Fever, particularly with neutropenia
- Abdominal pain
- Recent treatment
- Signs of dehydration.

REFERENCES

1. Siegel RL, Miller KD, Jemal A. Cancer statistics, 2017. CA Cancer J Clin 2017; 67(1):7–30.
2. Howlader N, Noone AM, Krapcho M, et al, editors. SEER cancer statistics review, 1975-2014. Bethesda (MD): National Cancer Institute; 2017. Available at: https://seer.cancer.gov/csr/1975_2014/. based on November 2016 SEER data submission, posted to the SEER web site.
3. Fragkandrea I, Nixon JA, Panagopoulou P. Signs and symptoms of childhood cancer: a guide for early recognition. Am Fam Physician 2013;88(3):185–92.
4. Mickley ME, Gutierrez C, Carney M. Oncologic and hematologic emergencies in children. In: Tintinalli JE, Stapczynski J, Ma O, et al, editors. Tintinalli's emergency medicine: a comprehensive study guide. New York: McGraw-Hill; 2016. p. 958–76 [Chapter 143].

5. Alakel N, Middeke JM, Schetelig J, et al. Prevention and treatment of tumor lysis syndrome, and the efficacy and role of rasburicase. Onco Targets Ther 2017;10: 597–605.
6. Lam JC, Chui CH, Jacobsen AS, et al. When is a mediastinal mass critical in a child? An analysis of 29 patients. Pediatr Surg Int 2004;20(3):180–4.
7. Bajciova V. Pediatric oncology: superior vena cava syndrome. In: Bajciova V, editor. Pediatric oncology. Brno (Czechia): Institute of Biostatistics and Analyses of Masaryk University. Available at: http://telemedicina.med.muni.cz/pediatric-oncology/index.php?pg=emergencies-in-pediatric-oncology–superior-vena-cava-syndrome. Accessed November 21, 2017.
8. Freedman JL, Rheingold SR. Management of oncologic emergencies. In: Lanzkowsky P, Lipton JM, Fish JD, editors. Lanzkowsky's manual of pediatric hematology and oncology. New York: Elsevier Inc; 2016. p. 605–19 [Chapter 32].
9. Sisk BA, Bluebond-Langner M, Wiener L, et al. Prognostic disclosures to children: a historical perspective. Pediatrics 2016;138(3).
10. Howard SC, Jones DP, Pui CH. The tumor lysis syndrome. N Engl J Med 2011; 364(19):1844–54.
11. Fox S. Neutropenic fever — Pediatric EM Morsels. Pediatric EM Morsels; 2017.
12. Rodrigues FG, Dasilva G, Wexner SD. Neutropenic enterocolitis. World J Gastroenterol 2017;23(1):42–7.
13. Kuiken NS, Rings EH, Tissing WJ. Risk analysis, diagnosis and management of gastrointestinal mucositis in pediatric cancer patients. Crit Rev Oncol Hematol 2015;94(1):87–97.
14. Al-Gwaiz LA, Babay HH. The diagnostic value of absolute neutrophil count, band count and morphologic changes of neutrophils in predicting bacterial infections. Med Princ Pract 2007;16(5):344–7.

Rapid Fire: Central Nervous System Emergencies

Sarah B. Dubbs, MD[a],*, Akilesh P. Honasoge, MD[b,c]

KEYWORDS

- Cancer • Metastases • Malignant spinal cord compression • Cauda equina
- Neurologic • Emergency

KEY POINTS

- A central nervous system emergency must be suspected in any patient with known cancer diagnosis and new neurologic symptoms or signs.
- The decision to image the brain or spine is dependent on finding key historical and examination features.
- When evaluating for spinal involvement, the preferred diagnostic examination is MRI of the entire spine.
- Therapeutic options include corticosteroids, radiation, and surgery, and should be discussed with the interdisciplinary oncology team.

CASE 1: LOWER EXTREMITY WEAKNESS AND FALLS
Pertinent History

A 51-year-old homeless man with a history of alcohol abuse presents after a fall. The patient is well-known to the emergency department and has been seen frequently for acute alcohol intoxication. On this presentation he was found by emergency medical services personnel on the sidewalk with a head injury. The patient reports that he does not remember the circumstances surrounding his head injury. He reports he has had many falls recently and often has difficulty with balance. He reports worsening bladder incontinence over the past month. He denies any other genitourinary complaints. The

Disclosure Statement: The authors have no relationship with a commercial company that has a direct financial interest in subject matter or materials discussed in article or with a company making a competing product.
[a] Department of Emergency Medicine, University of Maryland School of Medicine, 110 South Paca Street, 6th Floor, Suite 200, Baltimore, MD 21201, USA; [b] Department of Emergency Medicine, University of Maryland Medical Center, 110 South Paca Street, 6th Floor, Suite 200, Baltimore, MD 21201, USA; [c] Department of Internal Medicine, University of Maryland Medical Center, 110 South Paca Street, 6th Floor, Suite 200, Baltimore, MD 21201, USA
* Corresponding author.
E-mail address: sdubbs@som.umaryland.edu

patient reports worsening back pain over the past few months, but denies any specific trauma to the region.

PMH: Denies.

PSH: Appendectomy at age 13 years.

SH: Daily alcohol abuse for the past 15 years. 30 pack-year history of tobacco smoking. Denies any illicit drug use.

FMH: Hypertension, diabetes, heart attack, stroke, cancer (unknown type).

Medications: None.

Physical Examination

T: 36.8, BP: 165/110, HR: 91, RR:16, SpO$_2$: 92% on room air.

General: Alert and oriented ×3, disheveled appearing, smells of urine.

HEENT: Small hematoma to the left parietal scalp, mild abrasions to the area without active bleeding. Pupils equal, round, and reactive to light, poor oral dentition, mucous membranes dry.

Neck: Full range of motion, no midline cervical spine tenderness.

Cardiovascular: Regular rate and rhythm, no murmurs/rubs/gallops.

Pulmonary: Clear to auscultation bilaterally.

Abdominal: Soft, nontender, nondistended, normal bowel sounds.

Back: Tenderness to palpation over the lumbar spine.

Neurologic: 5/5 strength of bilateral upper extremities, 3/5 strength of bilateral lower extremities.

Diminished saddle sensation. Rectal tone diminished.

Finger-to-nose intact. Heel-to-shin abnormal bilaterally.

Diminished reflexes bilaterally in the lower extremities.

Musculoskeletal: Normal pulses throughout, full ROM of all extremities, no significant peripheral edema.

Laboratory Testing

CBC: Normal.

CMP: Normal.

Imaging

Computed tomography (CT) of the head without contrast: Small contusion to the soft tissue of the left posterior scalp, mild diffuse atrophy, normal ventricle size, otherwise normal.

CT lumbar spine without contrast: Mild L3 disc protrusion without significant stenosis, age-related diminished bone density, no acute fractures, otherwise normal.

Clinical Course

Based on clinical suspicion for cauda equina syndrome, the patient was given 10 mg of dexamethasone intravenously. Neurosurgery was consulted and a Foley catheter was placed for urinary retention. An emergent MRI showed a soft tissue tumor in the lumbar spinal canal causing acute compression of the cauda equina.

LEARNING POINTS
Introduction and Background

1. Cord compression is defined as compression in the dural sac and its contents by an extradural or intradural mass leading to neurologic damage. Malignant spinal cord compression (MSCC), is one of the most devastating neurologic complications of cancer, and constitutes an oncologic emergency. It affects 5% to 10%

of patients with cancer,[1,2] with the majority of cases resulting from spine metastases with extension to the epidural space.
2. Vertebral metastases, with or without spinal compression, causes pain and diminishes quality of life. As it progresses to compress the spine, patients suffer from voiding and defecation abnormalities, weakness, inability to ambulate, paralysis, sensory changes, and other neurologic deficits.
3. The cancers most commonly accounting for MSCC are breast, prostate, lung, and lymphoma. The disease-specific incidence of spinal cord compression is greatest in multiple myeloma, prostate, nasopharyngeal, and breast cancers.[3] Notably, 20% of newly diagnosed MSCC cases lack a history of cancer that time of diagnosis.[4]
4. Mak and colleagues[5] found that, from 1998 and 2016, American patients with cancer overall had a 3.4% annual incidence of MSCC requiring hospitalization, with a trend toward increased costs of hospitalization.

Physiology and Pathophysiology

1. Anatomy: The spinal cord extends from the base of the brain stem down to the conus medullaris at approximately the L1 or L2 vertebrae. Further down, the spinal cord becomes a series of spinal nerve roots called the cauda equina (Latin for *horse's tail*; **Fig. 1**).
   • Compression of any portion of the spinal cord can cause an acute epidural spinal cord compression syndrome.
   • Symptoms vary according to location of compression
2. Mechanisms of cord compression in MSCC
   • Direct extension of tumor into the epidural space from hematologic spread.
   • Pathologic fracture of a vertebral body that has been infiltrated by malignant cells. The bony fragments or resulting spinal instability causes mass effect on the spinal cord.
   • Intradural masses such as meningiomas, nerve sheath tumors, and leptomeningeal metastases may cause mass effect on the spinal cord.
   • Rarely, aggressive paravertebral tumors such as a Pancoast lung tumor will invade the epidural space directly.
3. Nonmetastatic but cancer-related causes of spinal cord compression include:
   • Epidural hematoma in patients with cancer-related coagulopathy; and
   • Abscess in immunocompromised patients.

Making the Diagnosis

1. The development of malignant spinal axis involvement and cord compression is a slow and insidious process. Pain and other symptoms are often attributed to other benign causes, especially if the patient does not carry a cancer diagnosis. It is imperative that emergency physicians obtain a thorough and directed history as well as perform a detailed physical examination to make the diagnosis, because the decision to image and investigate further depends on finding key historical and examination features.
2. Symptoms and signs
   • The most common presenting symptom for MSCC is pain. Any back pain in patients with cancer should be considered of metastatic origin until proven otherwise.
      i. Pain that worsens at night or with recumbence should raise red flags for spinal involvement.

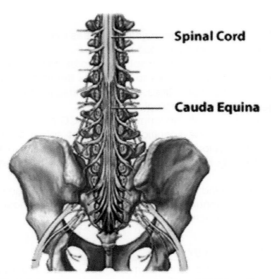

Fig. 1. Lower spinal cord anatomy. (*From* Lower spinal cord. Wikimedia commons. Available at: https://commons.wikimedia.org/wiki/File:Onurğa_beyni_at_quyruğu.jpg. Accessed March 30, 2018.)

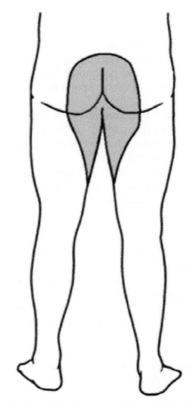

Fig. 2. Saddle anesthesia. (*From* Saddle anesthesia. Wikimedia commons. Available at: https://commons.wikimedia.org/wiki/File:Saddle_anesthesia.png. Accessed March 30, 2018.)

    ii. Early in the course, pain may be localized to the affected spinal segment with tenderness to percussion of the vertebral body.

    iii. Pain owing to epidural mass effect often presents with pain that is aggravated by sneezing, coughing, or other Valsalva maneuvers.

    iv. Involvement of the nerve roots causes symptoms with radicular qualities — sharp, shooting pain exacerbated by Valsalva maneuvers. This quality particularly makes the presentation easily mistaken for other more benign conditions.

- Symptoms of *neurogenic bladder dysfunction* may be overlooked or rationalized by patients and must be addressed in a direct manner when obtaining a history. Symptoms can range from hesitancy, nocturia, urinary retention, and incontinence.
- Only one-third of patients report lower extremity *weakness* as an initial symptom; however at diagnosis, less than one-third of patients are ambulatory.[1] Examination should include isolated strength testing of muscle groups, especially those innervated by the distal spinal cord roots.
- Few patients report *diminished sensation* at initial presentation, but in the case of intraneural tumor involvement, neuropathic features such as hyperalgesia and allodynia may predominate.[1] Sensory deficits with saddle anesthesia (**Fig. 2**) are noted often in cauda equina compression.[6]
- Regarding examination of deep tendon reflexes, compression of the more central conus medullaris can develop hyperreflexia, while diminished reflexes is more common with cauda equina syndrome.

3. Imaging

- Imaging should be guided by the history and examination. In general, emergent testing for MSCC should be triggered by patients presenting with back pain and concerning symptoms or signs (as detailed elsewhere in this article).
- Plain radiographs of the spine lack sensitivity and are not very valuable in this subset of patients.
- A CT scan can be helpful in showing osseous involvement; however, a negative CT scan has a poor negative predictive value for epidural or leptomeningeal involvement.
- The best diagnostic scan is MRI, which best shows the spinal cord and soft tissue masses, and is the most sensitive diagnostic test when MSCC is suspected in a patient with cancer.[1]

    i. Imaging of the entire spine should be obtained, because multiple levels of involvement present in up to one-third of patients.[7] Additionally, discrepancy in symptom level of up to 10 levels above or below the lesion has been described in the literature.[8]

    ii. The MRI should be obtained with gadolinium contrast enhancement, which allows for better characterization of the masses and allows metastases to be distinguished from other pathologic processes such as abscess and hematoma (see **Fig. 3**).

- An historical adjuvant to the CT scan is CT myelography, in which contrast dye is injected into the intrathecal space.[9] This diagnostic procedure was the gold standard of diagnosis in the pre-MRI era, and is only rarely used, except in those patients with contraindications to MRI.
- An important pitfall to note is relying on previous PET scans to rule out spine involvement. PET scans are screening tools and should never supersede clinical judgment in oncologic patients presenting with back pain or neurologic deficits.

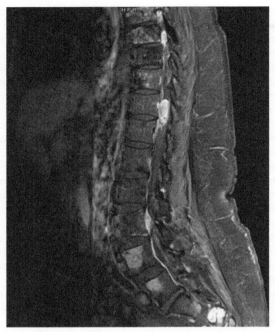

Fig. 3. This view of the thoracic and lumbar spine on a gadolinium-enhanced MRI shows multifocal osseous and epidural metastatic disease with spinal cord compression, including spinal cord/conus medullaris edema secondary to compression by a large T11 to T12 meta-static deposit.

Treating the Patient

1. The acute treatment in the emergency department consists of steroid administration, coordination with multiple consultants, and admission for inpatient care.
2. Corticosteroids
    - Randomized, controlled trials suggest that corticosteroids are beneficial as an adjunctive therapy in MSCC with the goals of improved pain control and reduction of vasogenic cord edema.[10,11]
        i. Commonly, dexamethasone is used with an initial bolus dose of 16 mg orally or intravenously, followed by up to 10 mg every 6 hours.
        ii. High-dose protocols have been studied, but it remains unclear if there are improved neurologic outcomes despite improved pain control.[12,13] Additionally, complications such as gastric ulcer, hallucinations, and insomnia are more likely with higher doses.[14]
        iii. If the primary cancer diagnosis is unknown and lymphoma is suspected, steroids may impact tissue diagnosis.[15] The decision to administer steroids in this case should be discussed with oncology.
3. Radiotherapy and surgery
    - There are multiple different neurosurgical and radiation therapies available, and the options available depend on numerous factors, including acuity, radiosensitivity of the tumor, and availability of resources.
    - No one therapy has shown clear superiority, with benefits often seen when they are used together.[16]

- Emergency physicians should ensure that radiation oncology and spine surgeons are urgently consulted to review and make recommendations on treatment.
4. Palliative and comfort care only
    - MSCC can be debilitating and carries a morbid average life expectancy for the patients diagnosed with it. Patients may opt for comfort care without interventions after overall prognosis and options are discovered and discussed by their oncologist and care team.

Case Conclusion

The spinal axis mass raised concern for malignancy in the patient. He was treated with steroids, admitted to the hospital, and taken for emergent radiation therapy. Further imaging revealed a lung mass and other areas suspicious for metastases. Subsequent biopsy confirmed the diagnosis of metastatic lung cancer.

CASE 2: NEW-ONSET SEIZURE

A 61-year-old woman is brought to the emergency department by ambulance after having a generalized tonic-clonic seizure at work. She has a reported history of hypertension and diabetes. Her finger-stick glucose obtained at the scene was 121 mg/dL. She is postictal and cannot provide further history.

Pertinent History

PMH: Hypertension, diabetes.
  SH: Unknown.
  FMH: Unknown.
  Medications: Unknown.

Physical Examination

T: 36.0, BP: 153/85, HR: 99, RR:17, SpO$_2$: 99% on room air.
  General: Drowsy, confused, mumbles incoherently in response to stimulus.
  HEENT: No external signs of trauma. Pupils equal, round, and reactive to light, mucous membranes dry.
  Neck: Full range of motion, no bruit.
  Cardiovascular: Regular rate and rhythm, no murmurs/rubs/gallops.
  Pulmonary: Clear to auscultation bilaterally.
  Abdominal: Soft, nontender, nondistended, normal bowel sounds.
  Neurologic: Drowsy, eyes open to voice. Mumbles incoherently, localizes painful stimulus. No facial asymmetry. Moves all extremities spontaneously with equal strength grossly.
  Musculoskeletal: Normal pulses throughout, full ROM of all extremities, no significant peripheral edema.
  Electrocardiogram: Normal sinus rhythm with normal axis and no signs of ischemia, or dysrhythmia.

Laboratory Testing

CBC: Normal.
  CMP: Normal.

Imaging

CT Head: Noncontrast CT of the head showed a large left parietal mass with some surrounding edema, but no hydrocephalus (**Fig. 4**A).

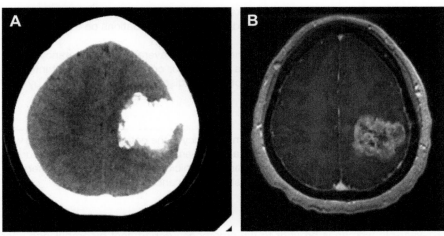

Fig. 4. (*A*): Noncontrast computed tomography scan shows a large left parietal mass. (*B*) T1-weighted image of a gadolinium-enhanced brain MRI showing the same mass.

Clinical Course

Neurosurgery was consulted immediately after the CT. The patient was started on an antiepileptic drug. Her mental status improved over a course of a few hours and she was admitted for further management.

LEARNING POINTS
Introduction and Background

1. Complications with intracranial masses, whether from primary brain malignancies or metastatic lesions, represent a large number of central nervous system–related cancer emergencies. These complications include vasogenic edema, hemorrhage, hydrocephalus, and seizures.
2. Brain metastasis occurs in 30% to 40% of cancers, most frequently originating from lung (50%) and breast (15%–25%) tumors.[17,18] These represent the most common neurologic complication of cancer.
3. Primary brain tumors (malignant and nonmalignant)
   - Overall average age of onset: 54 years.[19]
   - Most primary central nervous system tumors have a higher incidence rate in males,[20] but the major exception is meningiomas which are more common in females.
   - Most common types: Meningioma (36%), pituitary tumors (16%), glioblastoma (15%), vestibular schwannoma (8%), other astrocytoma (6%), and lymphoma (2%).[20]

Physiology and Pathophysiology

1. Complications of malignant intracranial masses arise mainly owing to mass effects of the tumors themselves and vasogenic edema that arises from the cytotoxic milieu around the tumor.
2. Hydrocephalus may result from a number of mechanisms:
   - Subependymal or leptomeningeal masses can block spinal fluid flow causing obstructing hydrocephalus; and
   - Decreased reabsorption of spinal fluid owing to the cancer can cause communicating hydrocephalus.

3. Hemorrhage can occur, especially in patients with cancer-related coagulopathy.
4. Venous thromboembolism is common in patients with brain tumors and the risk is correlated with higher grade malignancies. Venous thromboembolism develops in 30% of patients with high-grade glioma and in 20% of patients brain metastasis and central nervous system lymphoma.[21]
   - The increased hypercoagulability is believed to be related to the upregulation of tissue factor production. Tissue factor is a strong procoagulant that interacts with factor VII to initiate coagulation. It is also influences oncogenic signaling mechanisms that are involved in progression of the cancer.
   - In patients with brain tumors, the risk of anticoagulation causing intracranial hemorrhage complicates the treatment of venous thromboembolism when it develops.
5. The pathophysiologic mechanism for seizures related to brain tumors to this day is not clear.

Making the Diagnosis

1. If a patient with known cancer diagnosis presents with headache and new neurologic symptoms or signs, the emergency physician must consider brain involvement.
2. Symptoms and signs
   - Headache
     i. Headache is the most common symptom associated with brain tumors.
     ii. The classical description of a brain tumor associated headache is poorly supported by evidence, but has been described as tension type, dull, constant, exacerbated by Valsalva maneuvers, and is worse at night or in the early morning.
   - Seizures
     i. There is a high frequency of new-onset epilepsy as a presenting symptom of a brain tumor before radiologic diagnosis.[21,22]
        1. About 50% in high-grade gliomas.
        2. About 80% in low-grade gliomas.
        3. A diagnosis of seizure during the course of a neoplastic illness may portend a worse overall prognosis.
     ii. The most common presenting seizure in a brain tumor is a focal seizure.
     iii. Clinical manifestations of focal seizures vary depending on tumor location.
        1. Frontal: Focal tonic-clonic movements.
        2. Temporal: Sudden behavioral changes.
        3. Occipital: Visual disturbances.
   - Other symptoms and signs of intracranial mass include focal motor weakness, sensory disturbance, cranial nerve deficit, speech and coordination difficulties, nausea/vomiting, and altered mental status.
3. Imaging
   - CT imaging is a good initial screening tool because it is widely available and quick to obtain. Contrast enhancement does improve sensitivity of the test.
   - Gadolinium-enhanced MRI, however, is the true diagnostic modality of choice with higher sensitivity and specificity compared with CT for determining the number, size, and distribution of lesions.[22,23]
   - Although the vast majority of nonmalignant tumors are located in either the meninges or the pituitary, malignant tumors have a wider area of distribution: frontal lobe (23%), temporal lobe (17%), parietal lobe (11%), cerebellum (5%), meninges (2%), and pituitary (0.4%).[20]

Treating the Patient

1. *Corticosteroids* are used frequently to decrease brain edema in patients with signs of increased intracranial pressure. As discussed for MSCC, steroids should be avoided if new-onset lymphoma is highly suspected because it can decrease the sensitivity of cell diagnosis.
2. The role of *anticonvulsants* in patients with brain metastases has very limited class I evidence, but in general, most guidelines indicate that patients who are symptomatic with seizures should be treated with anticonvulsant drugs. Prophylactic anticonvulsants are not recommended in patients with brain metastases who have not had a seizure.
3. Stereotactic and whole-brain *radiotherapy* is applied in select patients in conjunction with radiation oncology specialists.
4. *Surgery* can be appropriate for some cases and can provide immediate relief of mass effect.

Case Conclusion

The patient underwent MRI to further elucidate the mass seen on CT imaging (**Fig. 4**B). The mass was ultimately diagnosed as a meningioma, and pathology revealed that it was malignant, which is extremely rare for this type of tumor.

DISCUSSION

Spinal cord compression and intracranial masses are two of the most devastating neurologic complications of cancer. They affect both life expectancy and quality of life. They are also difficult to diagnose early, especially when they are the presenting symptoms of a malignancy. The astute emergency physician can make a difference in patient's lives by paying close attention to the early symptoms of these complications, knowing when to trigger a more extensive diagnostic workup among the fray of patients presenting with otherwise very common complaints.

Pattern recognition

MSCC

- New back pain plus cancer.
- Pain aggravated by recumbence.
- Urinary retention, incontinence, saddle anesthesia, and extremity weakness.

Intracranial mass

- Persistent headache, worse with Valsalva maneuvers.
- Known cancer plus new headache and/or neurologic symptoms/signs.

REFERENCES

1. Becker KP, Baehring JM. Spinal cord compression. In: Devita VT Jr, Lawrence TS, Rosenberg SA, editors. Cancer principles and practice of oncology. 10th edition. Philadelphia: Wolters Kluwer Health; 2015. p. 1816–21.
2. Klimo P Jr, Thompson CJ, Kestle JR, et al. A meta-analysis of surgery versus conventional radiotherapy for the treatment of metastatic spinal epidural disease. Neuro Oncol 2005;7:64–76.

3. Loblaw DA, Laperriere NJ, Mackillop WJ. A population-based study of malignant spinal cord compression in Ontario. Clin Oncol (R Coll Radiol) 2003;15: 211–7.

4. Schiff D, O'Neill BP, Suman VJ. Spinal epidural metastasis as the initial manifestation of malignancy. Neurology 1997;49:452–6.

5. Mak KS, Lee LK, Mak RH, et al. Incidence and treatment patterns in hospitalizations for malignant spinal cord compression in the United States, 1998–2006. Int J Radiat Oncol Biol Phys 2011;80(3):824–31.

6. Helweg-Larson S, Sorenson PS. Symptoms and signs in metastatic spinal cord compression: a study of progression from first symptom until diagnosis in 153 patients. Eur J Cancer 1994;30A(3):396–8.

7. Hardy JR, Huddart R. Spinal cord compression- what are the treatment standards? Clin Oncol (R Coll Radiol) 2002;14:132–4.

8. Levack P, Graham J, Collie D, et al. Don't wait for a sensory level—listen to the symptoms: a prospective audit of the delays in diagnosis of malignant cord compression. Clin Oncol (R Coll Radiol) 2002;14:472–80.

9. Hagenau C, Grosh W, Currie M, et al. Comparison of spinal magnetic resonance imaging and myelography in cancer patients. J Clin Oncol 1987; 5(10):1663–9.

10. Klimo P Jr, Kestle JR, Schmidt MH. Treatment of metastatic spinal epidural disease: a review of the literature. Neurosurg Focus 2003;15:E1.

11. L'Espérance S, Vincent F, Gaudreault M, et al. Comité de l'évolution des pratiques en oncologie. Treatment of metastatic spinal cord compression: cepo review and clinical recommendations. Curr Oncol 2012;19:e478–90.

12. Sorensen S, Helweg-Larsen S, Mouridsen H, et al. Effect of high-dose dexamethasone in carcinomatous metastatic spinal cord compression treated with radiotherapy: a randomised trial. Eur J Cancer 1994;30A:22–7.

13. Delattre JY, Arbit E, Rosenblum MK, et al. High dose versus low dose dexamethasone in experimental epidural spinal cord compression. Neurosurgery 1988;22: 1005–7.

14. Heimdal K, Hirschberg H, Slettebo H, et al. High incidence of serious side effects of high-dose dexamethasone treatment in patients with epidural spinal cord compression. J Neurooncol 1992;12:141–4.

15. Al-Qurainy R, Collis E. Metastatic spinal cord compression: diagnosis and management. BMJ 2016;353:i2539.

16. George R, Jeba J, Ramkumar G, et al. Interventions for the treatment of metastatic extradural spinal cord compression in adults. Cochrane Database Syst Rev 2008;(4):CD006716.

17. Suh JH, Chao ST, Peereboom DM, et al. Metastatic cancer to the brain. In: Devita VT Jr, Lawrence TS, Rosenberg SA, editors. Cancer principles and practice of oncology. 10th edition. Philadelphia: Wolters Kluwer Health; 2015. p. 1832–44.

18. Scoccianti S, Ricardi U. Treatment of brain metastases: review of phase III randomized controlled trials. Radiother Oncol 2012;102:168–79.

19. Wrensch M, Minn Y, Chew T, et al. Epidemiology of primary brain tumors: current concepts and review of the literature. Neuro Oncol 2002;4(4): 278–99.

20. Ostrom QT, Gittleman H, Fulop J, et al. CBTRUS statistical report: primary brain and central nervous system tumors diagnosed in the United States in 2008-2012. Neuro Oncol 2015;17(Suppl 4):iv1–62.

21. Jo JT, Schiff D, Perry JR. Thrombosis in brain tumors. Semin Thromb Hemost 2014 Apr;40(3):325–31.
22. Lote K, Stenwig AE, Skullerud K, et al. Prevalence and prognostic significance of epilepsy in patients with gliomas. Eur J Cancer 1998;34(1):98–102.
23. Schellinger PD, Meinck HM, Thron A. Diagnostic accuracy of MRI compared to CCT in patients with brain metastases. J Neurooncol 1999;44:275–81.

Rapid Fire: Hypercalcemia

Angela Irene Carrick, DO*, Holly Briann Costner, DO

KEYWORDS

- Hypercalcemia • Malignancy • Endocrine • Treatment • Emergency medicine
- Metabolic emergency

KEY POINTS

- Hypercalcemia is most commonly due to hyperparathyroidism and malignancy but can be caused by medications and supplements, other endocrine disorders, and rheumatic disease.
- The acuity of development and degree of calcium elevation determines the extent of symptoms, which range from asymptomatic to coma.
- Once identified, it is necessary to confirm true hypercalcemia because it can be altered by serum albumin levels and pH.
- Treatment will vary by patient presentation and may require only follow-up in an outpatient setting for asymptomatic hypercalcemia or intensive care unit admission with a multispecialty approach for the comatose patient.
- The mainstay for emergency treatment is intravenous fluid hydration. Medications affecting calcium release and uptake can be used to further augment the level.

CASE: ALTERED MENTAL STATUS

Pertinent history: A 60-year-old man presents to the emergency department (ED) with confusion, hallucinations, and general weakness. His wife states the patient has not been himself for the last 1 to 2 weeks. He has had episodes of hallucinations of little pink feet running around. He has associated anorexia and decreased oral intake with a history of a 20 pound (9 kg) weight loss in the last 2 months. He has recently been treated for dental pain with amoxicillin by his primary doctor. He had right ankle surgery 2 to 3 months ago for pin and plate removal in which the bone was described as mush. Since the surgery, the patient has been on a progressive decline. He also complains of atraumatic right shoulder pain.

Social History: former smoker, denies alcohol or drug use.
Past Medical History: HTN, kidney stone.
Past Surgical History: ankles bilateral, lithotripsy.
Medications: lisinopril and hydrochlorothiazide, hydrocodone.

Disclosure Statement: The authors have nothing to disclose.
Emergency Medicine Residency, Norman Regional Hospital, 901 North Porter, Norman, OK 73071, USA
* Corresponding author. 6750 Belmar Circle, Norman, OK 73071.
E-mail address: aicarrick@me.com

Emerg Med Clin N Am 36 (2018) 549–555
https://doi.org/10.1016/j.emc.2018.04.008
0733-8627/18/© 2018 Elsevier Inc. All rights reserved.

emed.theclinics.com

Pertinent physical examination: temperature 36.7°C, blood pressure 91 over 57, heart rate 103, RR 20, Oxygen Saturation 96% on room air.

General: drowsy but arousable to verbal stimuli. He answers questions with minimal assistance and follows commands.

HEENT: PERRL, tympanic membranes clear, gingival swelling near left lower molar, posterior pharynx appears normal.

Neck: supple and nontender without lymphadenopathy. No nuchal rigidity.

Respiratory: clear to auscultation without retractions.

Cardiovascular: regular rhythm with mild tachycardia.

Gastrointestinal: soft, nontender, no masses. Bowel sounds normal.

Neurologic: cranial nerves 2 to 12 grossly intact. Strength is 5 out of 5 in upper extremities and 4 out of 5 in lower extremities. Sensation intact bilaterally without dermatomal sparing. Grips are equal. Performs finger to nose testing without ataxia. Speech is slurred.

Skin: warm and dry without rash.

Musculoskeletal: the right shoulder is mildly tender anteriorly and with normal range of movement. He is unable to hold the right upper extremity up against gravity secondary to pain. No neuromuscular deficits of the upper and lower extremities.

DIAGNOSTIC TESTING
Imaging

Laboratory assessment: **Table 1.**

Computed tomography, head: total opacification of the sphenoid sinuses with some bony erosion.

Chest radiography: negative.

Electrocardiogram: sinus rhythm rate 92, PR 194, QRS 112, QTC 467, nonspecific T wave abnormality.

Clinical course: intravenous (IV) fluids and furosemide were initiated, and nephrology was consulted for the patient's profound hypercalcemia. He was admitted to the intensive care unit for further management.

Table 1
Diagnostic imaging laboratory assessment

Laboratory Assessment	Emergency department	Day 6
White blood cell count (WBC)	8.1 10*9/L	5.0
Hemoglobin	11.2 mmol/L	9.6
Sodium	126 mmol/L	130
Potassium	3.0 mmol/L	3.7
Creatinine	1.99 mg/dL	2.59
Glucose	118 mg/dL	101
Albumin	3.2 g/dL	2.6
Calcium	16.8 mg/dL	9.6
Magnesium	1.7 mg/dL	1.8
Drug screen	Opiates positive	—
Urinalysis	10–20 WBC moderate bacteria	—
Lumbar puncture	Negative	—

LEARNING POINTS: HYPERCALCEMIA
Introductory or Background

1. Emergency physicians will assuredly encounter patients with hypercalcemia. It is a common problem with rates in the general population of 1 out of 1,000[1] inpatients, with malignancy in up to 20% to 30%.[1,2] It accounts for about 0.6% of admissions to the hospital.[1]
2. Patients can present with a spectrum of symptoms ranging from being completely asymptomatic to confusion and coma. The degree of hypercalcemia correlates with the severity of the symptoms.[3] The calcium level is used to categorize the patient as mild, moderate, or severe (**Table 2**).[3] (From Harborside, Huntington, NY; with permission.)
3. Every patient with cancer who has hypercalcemia deserves attention and needs additional laboratory values addressed.[4]
   - The urgency of treatment depends on both the symptoms and the actual calcium level. Some patients will need only arrangements for follow-up and further diagnostic testing, whereas some will require emergent management in the hospital.

Pathologic or Pathophysiologic Causes

1. The most common causes of hypercalcemia are hyperparathyroidism and malignancy (approximately 90% of cases[5]); however, the differential diagnosis is lengthy.
4. Less common causes include drugs (thiazides; vitamin A or D; calcium supplements, including antacids; and lithium), granulomatous diseases (eg, sarcoidosis), thyrotoxicosis, immobilization, familial hypercalcemia, and Addison disease.[1,4]
5. The most common malignancies causing hypercalcemia are lung, multiple myeloma, and renal cell carcinoma.[5]
   - Hypercalcemia from malignancy is an unfavorable prognostic indicator. This usually indicates a large tumor or widespread metastases. It would be unusual to find significant hypercalcemia and not find the underlying cancer during a workup of the patient.[4]
   - Cancer-causing hypercalcemia is thought to be from either of the following mechanisms:
     - Abnormal release of hormones (parathyroid hormone-related peptide, activated vitamin D, and PTH)[1-3]

Table 2
Signs and symptoms of hypercalcemia

	Mild (Corrected Calcium [CRC] 10.5–11.9 mg/dL)	Moderate (CRC 12.0–13.9 mg/dL)	Severe (CRC >14.0 mg/dL)
Neuropsychiatric	Anxiety, depression	Cognitive dysfunction	Lethargy, confusion, stupor, coma
Gastrointestinal	Anorexia, nausea, constipation	Anorexia, nausea, constipation	Pancreatitis
Renal	Polyuria	Dehydration	Renal insufficiency, dehydration
Cardiac	Shortened QT interval	Shortened QT interval	Arrhythmia, ventricular tachycardia
Musculoskeletal	None	Weakness	Weakness

Data from Inzucchi (2004); Ahrred & Hashiba (1988); and Kewiet, Ponssen, Janssens & Fels (2004). *From* Malangone S, Campen C. Hypercalcemia of malignancy. J Adv Pract Oncol 2015;6(6):588; with permission.

o The tumor's osteolytic activity in the bone (usually with multiple myeloma and cancers with multiple bony metastases).[1–3]

Making the Diagnosis

1. After finding an elevated serum calcium, the first step is to confirm true elevation.[2–4]
   - First the provider must check that the albumin level is normal. This is necessary because serum calcium level (bound plus unbound calcium) is greatly affected by the patient's albumin level. A large proportion of calcium is bound to albumin. The unbound (ie, ionized or free) calcium is what is active in the body. Therefore, a patient with low albumin who has a serum calcium level in the normal range could actually be hypercalcemic.[2,3]
   - Confirming hypercalcemia in the face of hypoalbuminemia can be done by applying the formula for corrected calcium (CRC) shown in **Box 1**.
   - An ionized serum calcium level can also be used to confirm the level of unbound calcium.
     o The ionized level, however, is greatly affected by the serum pH. The emergency provider is cautioned to interpret this level in context of the pH (**Box 2**).[2]
2. After confirming true hypercalcemia in the ED, the next steps for determining the cause and managing the patient occur simultaneously.
   - Additional studies commonly include a parathyroid hormone level (because hyperparathyroidism is 1 of the 2 main causes of hypercalcemia), a serum phosphorus (because hyperphosphatemia and hypophosphatemia is commonly found with hypercalcemia), and other specific hormone levels and diagnostic tests to evaluate for malignancy.[2–4]
   - The need for additional studies to be done in the ED will be determined by both the patient's disposition and the probable cause of the hypercalcemia.
3. Abnormal electrocardiogram findings that have been reported include
   - A shortened QT interval
   - Prolonged PR and QRS intervals
   - Flat or inverted T waves and the presence of a J wave following the QRS complex[6]

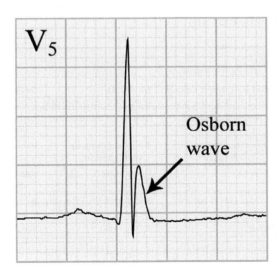

> **Box 1**
> **Calculating corrected calcium**
>
> CRC = serum calcium + 0.8 (4-serum albumin)
>
> *Data from* Malangone S, Campen C. Hypercalcemia of malignancy. J Adv Pract Oncol 2015;6(6):586–92; and Maier J, Levine S. Hypercalcemia in the intensive care unit: a review of pathophysiology, diagnosis, and modern therapy. J Intensive Care Med 2015;30(5):235–52.

- Scooped ST elevation similar to acute myocardial infarction can be seen, occuring most commonly in the anterior chest leads.[6]

Courtesy of Jason E. Roediger, CCT, CRAT; and https://commons.wikimedia.org/w/index.php?curid=19566138.

Treatment

1. Treatment depends on the severity and cause of the hypercalcemia, as well as the status of the patient.
   - Asymptomatic patients may only need arrangement for follow-up and further investigation.
   - Moderate to severely elevated calcium levels often require admission to the hospital for volume replacement and reduction of their calcium.
   - If malignancy is the primary cause of hypercalcemia, the main goal will be treating the cancer.[2]
2. IV fluid is the cornerstone of treatment in the ED. Fluid replaces the volume lost and promotes excretion of calcium.
   - Dehydration occurs due to nausea and poor oral intake, as well as the increased urine output that occurs from nephrogenic diabetes insipidus.[2]
   - The fluid of choice is isotonic saline.[2,4]
   - For moderate to severe dehydration, it is appropriate to give 1 to 2 L of fluid in the ED and then continue repletion in the hospital over the next few days.[2]
   - Exhibit caution with patients at risk for fluid overload, such as those with congestive heart failure or renal failure, or patients with cancer who have low albumin (who could develop third spacing).[2–4]
3. Calcitonin can be used for initial stabilization owing to its fairly quick onset of action. The combination of this medication with IV fluids can decrease calcium by 1 to 2 mg/dL in only a few hours.[4]
4. Bisphosphonates (pamidronate and zoledronic acid) work to lower calcium by inhibiting osteoclast activity in the bone, which causes resorption and subsequent calcium release into the blood. These take at least 48 hours to become effective and are used for long-term treatment.[2,4]
5. Denosumab is a new antiresorptive medication currently licensed only for osteoporosis but being used experimentally in severe hypercalcemia.[4] Studies show effectiveness in patients not responding to traditional bisphosphonates.[2]
6. Glucocorticoids have multiple mechanisms that help lower calcium by decreasing absorption by intestines, inhibiting resorption of bone,[2] and tumorolysis.[2] However,

> **Box 2**
> **pH and calcium**
>
> As pH decreases, calcium shifts from being albumin-bound to becoming ionized. Therefore, an alkalotic patient may have low ionized calcium and an acidotic patient may have a high ionized calcium level.[2]

these come with multiple potential complications.[3,4] They are mainly used to treat hypercalcemia from granulomatous diseases such as sarcoidosis, vitamin D toxicity, and hematologic malignancies.[4]

7. Furosemide is no longer recommended owing to risks of potential excessive diuresis and lack of beneficial supportive data.[4]

8. Withhold possible offending medications that may be causing hypercalcemia (eg, calcium, thiazides, lithium).

9. Dialysis can temporarily stabilize critical, comatose patients.[4]

CASE SUMMARY

Outcome: nephrology consulted and began furosemide and normal saline with replacement of potassium and magnesium. The patient was also started on pamidronate and calcitonin. Further workup and consultation with oromaxillofacial surgery and oncology revealed destructive bony lesions due to multiple myeloma, which resulted in his hypercalcemia. His altered mental state improved with resolution as the calcium returned to normal over a 6-day treatment period with IV hydration, furosemide, pamidronate, and calcitonin. The final diagnosis was hypercalcemia due to multiple myeloma with plasmacytosis. The patient was discharged to a skilled nursing facility on hospital day 36 with plans to begin chemotherapy in the outpatient setting.

CASE DISCUSSION

Hypercalcemia results in a constellation of symptoms that extends its effects throughout the body and mind. The phrase "bones, stones, moans, and groans" refers to musculoskeletal pain, kidney stones, mental status changes, and gastrointestinal upset. This is a commonly used mnemonic taught to medical students and residents to help them remember these symptoms. After a diagnosis of hypercalcemia is made, the underlying cause must be explored, most commonly leading to undiagnosed hyperparathyroid or malignancy as the cause. The main focus of treatment is initial correction of the elevated calcium with IV fluid hydration followed by medications to help modify calcium uptake and release.

Pattern recognition
• Bones, stones, moans, and groans
• Symptoms can be subtle (new psychiatric behavior, unexplained bone pain)
• Severity of symptoms correlates with level of calcium elevation
• Usually from hyperparathyroid and malignancy
• If albumin is low, use CRC formula
• Initial treatment isotonic saline

REFERENCES

1. Turner J. Hypercalcaemia—presentation and management. Clin Med 2017;17(3): 270–3.

2. Goldner W. Cancer-related hypercalcemia. J Oncol Pract 2016;12(5):426–32.

3. Malangone S, Campen C. Hypercalcemia of malignancy. J Adv Pract Oncol 2015; 6(6):586–92.

4. Maier J, Levine S. Hypercalcemia in the intensive care unit: a review of pathophysiology, diagnosis, and modern therapy. J Intensive Care Med 2015;30(5):235–52.
5. Naganathan S, Gossman WG. Hypercalcemia. StatPearls; 2017. Available at: http://www.ncbi.nlm.nih.gov/books/NBK430714/.
6. Durant E, Singh A. ST elevation due to hypercalcemia. Am J Emerg Med 2017; 35(7):1033.e3-6.

Rapid Fire: Pericardial Effusion and Tamponade

Akilesh P. Honasoge, MD[a,b], Sarah B. Dubbs, MD[a,*]

KEYWORDS

- Pericardial effusion • Cardiac tamponade • Cancer • Oncologic emergency
- Pericardiocentesis • Electrical alternans

KEY POINTS

- Suspect tamponade in patients with cancer presenting with tachycardia, shortness of breath, and hypotension.
- Look for low voltage and electrical alternans on electrocardiogram.
- Perform bedside echocardiogram early to diagnose pericardial effusion and/or tamponade.
- Use ultrasound guidance if possible during pericardiocentesis.
- Avoid intubation in patients with pericardial effusion or tamponade.

CASE: SHORTNESS OF BREATH, TACHYCARDIA, AND CANCER

Pertinent history: A 41-year-old man with recently diagnosed stage IV lung adenocarcinoma presents to the emergency department with shortness of breath. The patient was diagnosed 3 weeks prior with stage IV adenocarcinoma causing a complete occlusion of his right mainstem bronchus and a large malignant pleural effusion, which was treated with chest tube drainage. He reports he had been doing well after discharge but started having progressively worsening shortness of breath and dyspnea on exertion 24 hours later. He denies any fevers or chills. He reports mild chest pain only present with deep inspiration and coughing.

Past Medical History: stage IV lung adenocarcinoma after 2 rounds of thoracic radiation; plan to start systemic chemotherapy the following week.

Medications: none.

Disclosure Statement: The authors have no relationship with a commercial company that has a direct financial interest in the subject matter or materials discussed in the article or with a company making a competing product.

[a] Department of Emergency Medicine, University of Maryland Medical Center, 110 South Paca Street, 6th Floor, Suite 200, Baltimore, MD 21201, USA; [b] Department of Internal Medicine, University of Maryland School of Medicine, 110 South Paca Street, 6th Floor, Suite 200, Baltimore, MD 21201, USA

* Corresponding author.

E-mail address: sdubbs@som.umaryland.edu

Emerg Med Clin N Am 36 (2018) 557–565

https://doi.org/10.1016/j.emc.2018.04.004

0733-8627/18/© 2018 Elsevier Inc. All rights reserved.

emed.theclinics.com

Physical examination: Temperature: 37.1; blood pressure (BP): 155/105; heart rate: 128; Respiratory Rate = 28; oxygen saturation as measured by pulse oximetry: 82% on room air, 100% on Non-Rebreather

General: Alert, ill appearing in moderate respiratory distress, oriented × 3

Head/Eyes/Ears/Nose/Throat (HEENT): Pupils equal, round, and reactive to light, mucous membranes dry, no stridor

Neck: full range of motion (ROM), no significant Jugular venous distension but examination limited because of accessory muscle usage

Cardiovascular: regular rhythm, tachycardic, no murmurs/rubs/gallops, sinus tachycardia on the monitor

Pulmonary: significantly decreased lung sounds over right chest, coarse rhonchi throughout

Abdominal: soft, nontender, nondistended, normal bowel sounds

Neurologic: 5/5 strength and normal sensation throughout

Musculoskeletal: normal pulses throughout, full ROM of all extremities, no significant peripheral edema

Diagnostic testing	
WBC	10.3 K/mcL
Hgb	9.7 g/dL
Hct	29.4%
Plt	311 K/mcL
Na	135 mmol/L
Potassium	3.8 mmol/L
Cl	101 mmol/L
CO_2	23 mmol/L
Glucose	161 mg/dL
BUN	10 mg/dL
Creatinine	0.62 mg/dL
Calcium	9.3 mg/dL
Troponin	<0.02 ng/mL
Protime	18.1 s
INR	1.5
PTT	29 s

Abbreviations: BUN, serum urea nitrogen; Cl, chloride; CO_2, carbon dioxide; Hct, hematocrit; Hgb, hemoglobin; INR, international normalized ratio; Na, sodium; Plt, platelets; Protime, prothrombin time; PTT, partial thromboplastin time; WBC, white blood cell.

Electrocardiogram (EKG): As seen in **Fig. 1**, the EKG revealed sinus tachycardia and alternating QRS amplitude from beat to beat, also known as electrical alternans.

Portable chest radiography: A large right pleural effusion and enlarged cardiac silhouette was seen on portable anteroposterior chest film, as seen in **Fig. 2**.

Clinical course: A diagnostic workup was quickly initiated with the laboratory tests, EKG, and radiograph, as mentioned earlier and in **Figs. 1** and **2**. A bedside ultrasound was performed that showed a large pericardial effusion with a swinging motion of the

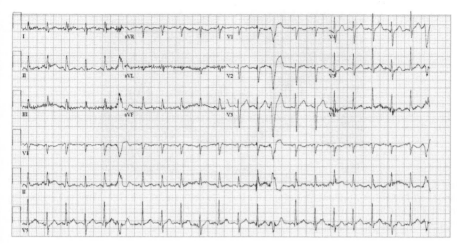

Fig. 1. EKG shows sinus tachycardia and electrical alternans.

patient's heart in the pericardial sac (**Fig. 3**). Closer inspection demonstrated right ventricular diastolic collapse raising concern for cardiac tamponade. Manual BP measurement demonstrates a drop in systolic BP by 20 mm Hg during inspiration (>10 mm Hg is suggestive of pulsus paradoxus and concerning for cardiac tamponade).

Cardiac surgery was contacted for a pericardial window. The patient was not intubated because of the concern for hemodynamic collapse from increased intrathoracic pressure. The BP remained stable.

Over the next 30 minutes, as the operating room was prepared, the patient became increasingly diaphoretic and somnolent. Repeat BP was 77/35. An emergent

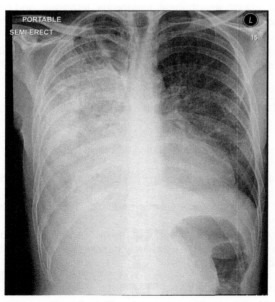

Fig. 2. Portable anteroposterior chest film demonstrates large right pleural effusion and enlarged cardiac silhouette.

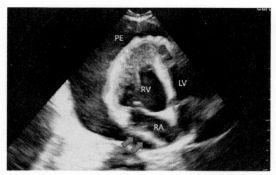

Fig. 3. A large pericardial effusion is seen on this 2-dimensional apical view during echocardiogram. The heart appears globular, and there is collapse of the right atrium (*arrows*) in this still image taken during early ventricular diastole. LV, left ventricle; PE, pericardial effusion; RA, right atrium; RV, right ventricle.

pericardiocentesis was performed yielding about 100 mL of bloody fluid with immediate return of BP to 140 systolic. The patient was then emergently taken to the operating room with a pericardial window yielding an additional 400 mL of blood in the pericardial sac with complete stabilization of the patient's hemodynamics.

LEARNING POINTS
Introduction and Background

1. Pericardial effusion in oncologic patients is most commonly caused by contiguous extension from a local primary tumor, metastases seeding the pericardium, or inflammation due to either radiation or an idiopathic cause.
   - The most common types of cancer associated with malignant pericardial effusion are lung, breast, esophageal, melanoma, leukemia, and lymphoma.
   - Rarely, mesothelioma, fibrosarcoma, and lymphangioma can be the cause of primary pericardial cancers.
2. Overall, malignant pericardial effusion occurs in approximately 10% of all patients with cancer, and about 33% of all these patients will die as a result of this involvement.[1]

Physiology/Pathophysiology

1. Malignant cells that have invaded the parietal/fibrous pericardium disrupt the normal homeostatic mechanisms that maintain the appropriate amount of pericardial fluid.[2]
2. Mediastinal involvement and radiation therapy also disrupt pericardial fluid homeostasis.
3. Patients with cancer may also develop increased fibrosis of the pericardium, making it more constrictive.
4. The increased volume and/or a fibrotic pericardium then leads to elevated pressures within the pericardial space.
5. Tamponade occurs when the pressure of the pericardial fluid exceeds the diastolic filling pressure of the right heart, ultimately decreasing cardiac output and causing obstructive shock.

Making the Diagnosis

1. Malignant pericardial effusions develop insidiously. Symptoms, therefore, are insidious and vague until full tamponade physiology ensues.

2. Presenting symptoms most often include the following:
   - Dyspnea
   - Fatigue
   - Generalized weakness
   - Dizziness or lightheadedness
3. Once the effusion evolves into tamponade, patients or their families will report the following:
   - Palpitations
   - Orthopnea
   - Respiratory distress
   - Altered mentation
4. Vital sign abnormalities may include the following:
   - Tachypnea
   - Tachycardia
   - Hypotension
   - Narrowed pulse pressure (often-overlooked).
5. Significant physical examination findings include the following:
   - Decreased or muffled heart sounds
   - Distended neck veins
   - Beck's triad (muffled heart sounds, distended neck veins, and hypotension, is only present in a minority of patients with pericardial tamponade).[3]
   - Pulsus paradoxus
     a. Often described in the literature regarding signs of cardiac tamponade, it is defined by a systolic BP drop of more than 10 mm Hg during respiratory inspiration.
     b. In one study, among medical causes of cardiac tamponade, pulsus paradoxus was present in about 98% of cases even in the absence of hypotension.[4]
     c. Pulsus paradoxus is traditionally gauged using a manual BP and noting Korotkoff during the respiratory cycle; however, this method may be cumbersome and inefficient, especially in unstable emergency department patients.[5,6]
     d. Similar observations can be made, however, by observing an arterial line pulse pressure wave or by palpating the patients' pulse during the respiratory cycle. In hemodynamically unstable patients, assessment for pulsus paradoxus should not delay more definitive testing, such as cardiac ultrasound.[7]
6. **Fig. 4** summarizes the evolution of symptoms and examinations findings in pericardial effusion and tamponade.
7. The classic EKG findings of cardiac tamponade (**Fig. 5**) are as follows below. Argula and colleagues[8] studied a population with known malignant pericardial effusion and found that the presence of all 3 EKG findings had a 100% positive predictive value for tamponade.
   - Tachycardia
   - Low voltage
   - Electrical alternans
8. Radiographic findings can suggest pericardial effusion but are not diagnostic of tamponade.
   - On plain radiography of the chest, the cardiac silhouette appears enlarged and may be globular or like an old-fashioned water bottle.
   - A coexistent pleural effusion can be seen in a third of cases (decamp).
   - Computed tomography of the chest will more definitively diagnose a pericardial effusion but cannot assess for tamponade physiology.

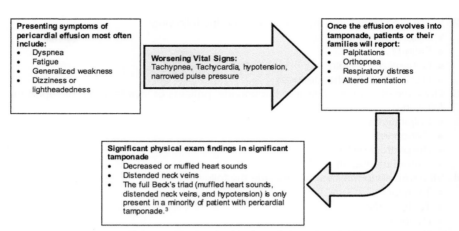

Presenting symptoms of pericardial effusion most often include:
- Dyspnea
- Fatigue
- Generalized weakness
- Dizziness or lightheadedness

Worsening Vital Signs:
Tachypnea, Tachycardia, hypotension, narrowed pulse pressure

Once the effusion evolves into tamponade, patients or their families will report:
- Palpitations
- Orthopnea
- Respiratory distress
- Altered mentation

Significant physical exam findings in significant tamponade
- Decreased or muffled heart sounds
- Distended neck veins
- The full Beck's triad (muffled heart sounds, distended neck veins, and hypotension) is only present in a minority of patient with pericardial tamponade.[3]

Fig. 4. Summary of the evolution of symptoms and examination findings in pericardial effusion and tamponade.

9. Ultrasound has become a vital tool in quick and effective bedside diagnosis of hypotensive and unstable patients.
   - Pericardial effusion and tamponade physiology can be reliably detected by the emergency physician using basic cardiac ultrasound windows.[9]
   - Tamponade on cardiac ultrasound or echocardiography appears as collapse of the right ventricle free wall during diastole. This collapse is sometimes described as the right cardiac free walls appearing to undulate in a serpentine pattern or, more subtly, move as if it is a trampoline with someone jumping on it.
   - The heart may also be observed to be swinging back and forth within the pericardial sac.

TREATING PATIENTS

1. The goal of treatment must be urgent relief of the increased pericardial pressure once tamponade is diagnosed or suspected.
2. Temporizing measures while setting up for pericardiocentesis
   - Provide supplemental oxygen by nasal cannula or nonrebreather.

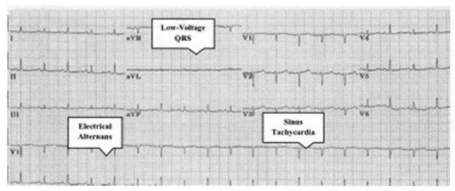

Fig. 5. The classic EKG signs of pericardial effusion. (*Courtesy of* Colin Kaide, MD, Columbus, Ohio, USA.)

    a. It should be noted that intubation or any positive pressure ventilation may induce or worsen tamponade in patients with pericardial effusion. The increased intrathoracic pressure decreases venous return and, thus, worsens the physiologic effects on cardiac output, leading to severe hemodynamic instability.[10]

    b. Proceed with caution if mechanical ventilation is unavoidable.

- Intravenous fluids may help temporize hypotension by expanding the intravascular volume.
- Vasopressors may also temporize hemodynamics while preparing for pericardiocentesis. Dobutamine and dopamine have been reported to improve hemodynamics in the setting of tamponade.[11] Norepinephrine and isoproterenol have shown improved hemodynamics in animal model studies but have not shown a benefit in human studies.[12,13]

3. Definitive treatment requires drainage via pericardiocentesis or surgical pericardial window.
- If possible, pericardiocentesis should be performed by an interventional cardiologist or cardiothoracic surgeon under fluoroscopy to prevent inadvertent perforation of the ventricular wall and to assist in drainage of potentially loculated effusions.
- In the case of unstable or crashing patients, the procedure should be performed by the emergency physician who is immediately available at the bedside.
- The ultrasound-guided approach is the safest and most reliable method for diagnosis and treatment of pericardial effusion and tamponade.[14] The landmark approach is associated with much higher rates of complication, such as puncture of the lung, ventricle, or coronary vessels.
- Aspiration of as little as 50 mL of fluid can significantly improve tamponade physiology.

4. Materials
- If a pericardiocentesis kit is not available, a central line or pigtail catheter kit can be used. If this is unavailable or the needle is not long enough, a long lumbar puncture needle can be used. The advantage of a central line kit is the ability to thread a wire into the pericardium and place a catheter for continued drainage, as even micropuncture kits often will not thread through a lumbar puncture needle.

5. Ultrasound-guided pericardiocentesis
- Elevate the head of the bed to 30° to 45° to bring the heart closer to the anterior chest wall.
- Cleanse the anterior and left lateral chest wall and upper abdomen with betadine or chlorhexidine.
- Making every effort to use aseptic technique, including using a sterile ultrasound probe cover and gel, locate the deepest pocket of pericardial fluid reachable by your needle using the apical, parasternal, and subxiphoid windows. The apical approach has been shown to be most effective; however, it does come with increased risk of pneumothorax.[15]
- After injecting local anesthesia, if time allows, insert the needle over the nearest rib toward and into the pericardial space, using the ultrasound in real time to confirm placement.

6. Landmark-guided pericardiocentesis
- Prepare the patient position and chest/abdominal wall as described earlier, and use standard aseptic precautions if time allows.
- Insert the needle 1 cm inferior to the subxiphoid or left sternocostal margin.
- Advance toward the left shoulder at a 30° to 45° angle, maintaining negative pressure on the syringe until pericardial fluid is obtained

Ultrasound-guided pericardiocentesis (preferred over landmark-guided technique)

- The deepest pocket of pericardial fluid reachable by needle drainage should be identified by ultrasound (usually apical).
- Insert the needle over the nearest rib toward and into the pericardial space using real-time ultrasound guidance.

Landmark-guided pericardiocentesis

- If using the blind approach, the needle should be inserted 1 cm inferior to the subxiphoid or left sternocostal margin and advanced toward the left shoulder at a 30 to 45° angle, maintaining negative pressure on the syringe.

CASE CONCLUSION

The patient's hospital course was complicated by the development of a pulmonary embolus, biventricular thrombus, and embolic stroke. Anticoagulation was difficult because of the persistent hemorrhagic drainage from his pericardium. With this worsening clinical condition and poor prognosis of the lung adenocarcinoma, he was eventually transitioned to comfort care and died.

DISCUSSION

Cardiac tamponade is easy to overlook in medical patients, as they often do not present with the classically described Beck triad. In oncologic patients, the vague and progressive symptoms are often attributed to the cancer itself. When evaluating tachypnea in patients at risk for a pericardial effusion, an EKG and bedside ultrasound can significantly aid diagnosis. The most difficult aspect of managing patients with pericardial tamponade who are not yet in cardiac arrest is making the decision as the emergency physician to proceed with an emergency department pericardiocentesis. This point is especially true when definitive treatment is in the hospital but not quite ready to intervene on the time schedule dictated by the circumstances. The procedure itself, especially in the era of bedside ultrasound, is simple in comparison with the diagnosis and decision to proceed with the pericardiocentesis.

Pattern recognition

Malignant pericardial effusion with tamponade
- Tachycardia, tachypnea, hypotension
- Beck triad: hypotension, dilated neck veins, muffled heart sounds; all 3 not always present
- EKG: low voltage and electrical alternans
- Echocardiogram: pericardial effusion, diastolic collapse of right atrium and/or right ventricle free wall
- Do not delay pericardiocentesis if hemodynamically unstable

REFERENCES

1. Maisch B, Ristic A, Pankuweit S. Evaluation and management of pericardial effusion in patients with neoplastic disease. Prog Cardiovasc Dis 2010;53(2):157–63.
2. DeCamp M, Mentzer S, Swanson S, et al. Malignant effusive disease of the pleura and pericardium. Chest 1997;112(4 Suppl):291S.
3. Sternbach G. Claude beck: cardiac compression triads. J Emerg Med 1988;6(5): 417–9.

4. Guberman BA, Fowler NO, Engel PJ, et al. Cardiac tamponade in medical patients. Circulation 1981;64:633–40.
5. Jay GD, Onuma K, Davis R, et al. Analysis of physician ability in the measurement of pulsus paradoxus by sphygmomanometry. Chest 2000;118:348–52.
6. Shim C, Williams MH Jr. Pulsus paradoxus in asthma. Lancet 1978;8063:530–1.
7. Mallemat HA, Tewelde SZ. Pericardiocentesis. In: Roberts JR, Custalow CB, Thomsen TW, editors. Roberts and Hedge's clinical procedures in emergency medicine. 6th edition. Philadelphia: Elsevier Saunders; 2014. p. 298–318.
8. Argula RG, Negi SI, Blanchs J, et al. Role of a 12-lead electrocardiogram in the diagnosis of cardiac tamponade as diagnosed by transthoracic echocardiography in patients with malignant pericardial effusion. Clin Cardiol 2015;38(3): 139–44.
9. Ghane MR, Gharic M, Ebrahimi A, et al. Accuracy of early rapid ultrasound in shock (RUSH) examination performed by emergency physician for diagnosis of shock etiology in critically ill patients. J Emerg Trauma Shock 2015;8(1):5–10.
10. Moller C, Schoonbee C, Rosendorff C. Haemodynamics of cardiac tamponade during various modes of ventilation. Br J Anaesth 1979;51:409.
11. Gabram SG, Devanney J, Jones D, et al. Delayed hemorrhagic pericardial effusion: case reports of a complication from severe blunt chest trauma. J Trauma 1992;32:794.
12. Martins JB, Manuel WJ, Marcus ML, et al. Comparative effects of catecholamines in cardiac tamponade; experimental and clinical studies. Am J Cardiol 1980;46:459.
13. Zhang H, Spapen H, Vincent JL. Effects of dobutamine and norepinephrine on oxygen availability in tamponade-induced stagnant hypoxia: a prospective, randomized, controlled study. Crit Care Med 1994;22:299.
14. Tsang TSM, Freeman WK, Sinak LG, et al. Echocardiographically guided pericardiocentesis: evolution and state-of-the-art technique. Mayo Clin Proc 1998;73:647.
15. Salem K, Mulji A, Lonn E. Echocardiographically guided pericardiocentesis—the gold standard for the management of pericardial effusion and cardiac tamponade. Can J Cardiol 1999;15:1251–5.

Rapid Fire: Sickle Cell Disease

Michael Porter, MD*

KEYWORDS

- Sickle cell disease • Acute chest syndrome • Aplastic crisis • Splenic sequestration
- Sickle cell anemia

KEY POINTS

- Sickle cell emergencies are most commonly related to acute anemia or vasoocclusive crisis.
- The cause of acute anemia must be differentiated between hemolytic, aplastic, or sequestration to determine treatment.
- Acute chest syndrome is the leading cause of morbidity and mortality in sickle cell disease. Early recognition and treatment are key.
- Sickle cell vasoocclusive diseases have many other presentations that require knowledge of presentation patterns and specific treatments.

CASE: FLULIKE SYMPTOMS

Pertinent history: A 29-year-old man with a history of sickle cell disease (SCD) presents to the emergency department (ED) with concerns over flulike symptoms. He works as a school teacher, and over the past week several of his students have developed influenza. Three days ago he developed some increasing soreness in his arms and legs. He first thought this was his sickle cell pain and treated it with his oxycodone that he is prescribed. However, over the past 2 days he has developed increasing cough productive of green sputum and chills. He reports pain in his chest, which he attributes to coughing spells. The chest pain causes him to have difficulty taking a deep breath. Today he developed shortness of breath at rest and decided to seek emergency care. He denies a sore throat, rhinorrhea, headache, or abdominal pain.

PHM: SCD.

Medications: hydroxyurea, oxycodone.

SH: occasional marijuana use, last 1 week ago, denies other drugs/tobacco/alcohol use.

Pertinent physical examination: Blood pressure 172/84, pulse 115, temperature 100.7°F, RR 26, peripheral capillary oxygen saturation 89%

Disclosure Statement: The author has no disclosures.
Department of Emergency Medicine, Norman Regional Hospital, Norman, OK, USA
* 409 Northwest 21st Street, Oklahoma City, OK 73103.
E-mail address: Michael.porter@okstate.edu

Emerg Med Clin N Am 36 (2018) 567–576
https://doi.org/10.1016/j.emc.2018.04.002
0733-8627/18/© 2018 Elsevier Inc. All rights reserved.

General: awake and alert; noted mild respiratory distress
HEENT: equal, round, pupils reactive to light; tympanic membranes normal bilaterally; nasal turbinates mildly edematous; normal oropharynx
Neck: supple, no JVD
Cardiovascular: tachycardic with regular rate; no murmur appreciated
Pulmonary: rales to right lower lung field; splinting with deep inspiration
Abdominal: abdomen soft and nondistended; bowel sounds normal; no hernias or masses appreciated
Neurologic: alert and oriented × 3; nonfocal throughout
Musculoskeletal: compartments soft, though pain from palpation in all 4 extremities; radial/ulnar and dorsal pedis pulses 3+ bilateral; normal strength and sensation × 4

Diagnostic findings	
WBC	15
HgB	9
Platelets	300
Reticulocyte count	3%
Na	138
K	3.9
Cl	100
CO_2	24
Glucose	128
ALT	28
AST	30
Bilirubin	1.1

Abbreviations: ALT, alanine aminotransferase; AST, aspartate aminotransferase; Cl, chloride; CO_2, carbon dioxide; HgB, hemoglobin; K, potassium; Na, sodium; WBC, white blood cell.

Chest radiograph (CXR): new right lower lobe infiltrate as compared with previous CXR; no pneumothorax; cardio-mediastinal silhouette normal in appearance.
Electrocardiogram: sinus tachycardia without acute ST depression or elevation.
Plan: aggressive pain management, gentle hydration, antibiotics, oxygen.
Patient's Course: The patient presented with concerns over catching the flu from his students. He has a history of SCD, and the provider was concerned about the possibility of worsening underlying pathology, such as acute chest syndrome. Vital signs demonstrated fever, tachycardia, and hypoxia. The patient had tachypnea as well, which was thought to be due to splinting from pain. After multiple rapid doses of intravenous (IV) hydromorphone, the patient's pain improved. He was placed on 3 L of oxygen by nasal cannula with improvement of hypoxia. His respiratory splinting decreased and his tachypnea resolved. Respiratory therapy was instructed to start the patient on incentive spirometry every hour. D5 1/4NS was administered at 200 mL/h. His hemoglobin (HgB) returned at 9 mg/dL, which the patient reported as close to his baseline hemoglobulin of 10 mg/dL. Rapid influenza swab was obtained and read as negative. Ceftriaxone and azithromycin were administered because of new infiltrate on CXR. Arterial blood gas (ABG) was obtained showing the following:

pH	7.31
P_{CO_2}	50
HCO_3	24
P_{O_2}	58
SaO_2	90%

Abbreviations: HCO_3, bicarbonate; SaO_2, oxygen saturation.

Although the patient's saturations had improved, his P_{O_2} was found to be low. The emergency provider contacted the patient's hematologist for a discussion of starting exchange transfusion. The hematologist agreed with this recommendation along with a plan for admission to the hospital.

LEARNING POINTS: SICKLE CELL DISEASE
Introductory/Background

1. Approximately 70,000 people in the United States have SCD. It affects predominantly equatorial African people groups, however, also occurs in Middle Eastern, Indian, and Mediterranean populations.[1] SCD occurs in 1 in 500 African American newborns, and the prevalence of the recessive gene (carrier state) occurs in about 8% of African Americans.
2. The formation of sickle-shaped red blood cells (RBCs) causes vasoocclusion and leads to a variety of complications that can cause morbidity and mortality in affected patients.[2]
   - Vasoocclusive pain crises are a common problem causing patients with SCD to seek treatment in the ED.
   - Acute chest syndrome is the leading cause of death of patients with SCD.[3]
   - Patients are at high risk for other embolic pathology, such as stroke, hepatic/splenic infarction, microvascular kidney disease, and venous thromboembolism.[4] Patients with SCD experience chronic anemia, which may lead to cardiomegaly.[5,6] They are also susceptible to acute anemia due to chronic anemia complicated by splenic sequestration, hemolysis, or aplastic crisis.

Physiology/Pathophysiology

1. SCD-SS (HbSS) is due to a mutation in the tetramer of the polypeptide chains in HgB. HgB A is the predominant (96%–98%) form of HgB in the adult body. It consists of 2 α-globin chains and 2 β-globin chains. The β-globin chain is mutated in SCD. Genetic mutations cause the formation of abnormal polypeptide in the β chain of the HgB molecule, producing HgB S. The mutation is a valine for glutamic acid substitution in the sixth position of the β-globin chain. Under hypoxic conditions, the HgB S polymerizes, changing shape and causing the cells to deform and become sickled in appearance.[7] Sickled RBCs tend to clump together, making the blood more viscous and causing microvascular occlusion. Sickled RBCs have an abnormally short life span, roughly 20 days, versus the 120-day life span of a normal RBC resulting in a chronic anemia.
2. SCD-SC (HbSC) is the second most common form of SCD, occurring in 25% of patients. It affects those with the S/C genotype in which one sickle gene mutation (HgB S) and one HgB C gene mutation are both inherited. As a result of the 2 similar gene defects, HbSC disease is associated with similar symptoms to HbSS disease (**Figs. 1** and **2**).

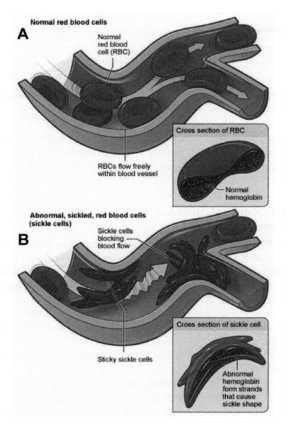

Fig. 1. Cross sections of blood cells. (*A*) Normal blood cells and (*B*) abnormal, sickled blood cells. (*From* National Heart, Lung, and Blood Institute. What is sickle cell anemia? Bethesda (MD): National Institutes of Health; 2008.)

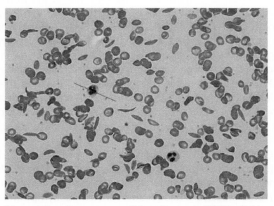

Fig. 2. Sickle cells. (*From* https://commons.wikimedia.org/wiki/File:Sickle_cells.jpg.)

Making the Diagnosis

SCD complications present in a variety of different ways to the ED. Making the diagnosis involves and understanding of the different varieties of pathology. Most complications will be related to either a vasoocclusive issue or anemia.[2] The first step to differentiating a sickle cell crisis is to determine if there is an acute anemic crisis. Most patients will know their baseline HbG, or it may be determined by review of the medical record.

1. Acute anemia: All patients with SCD have increased hemolysis and RBC destruction due to their condition and will usually be moderately anemic. A drop of 2 g/dL from baseline is considered acute.[7] The next step will be to differentiate between aplastic crisis or sequestration/hemolysis. To do this, obtain the reticulocyte count.
   - A low reticulocyte count indicates an aplastic crisis.
     - Bone marrow production is reduced, exacerbating chronic sickle cell anemia.
     - Eighty percent of cases are due to parvovirus B19 infection.[8] Less common causes include viruses, medications, and autoimmune disorders.
     - It is more common in children than adults.
   - There is a high reticulocyte count.
     - Sequestration is as follows:
       a. Most commonly the spleen sequesters RBCs. Less commonly the liver can sequester RBCs.[9]
       b. Splenic sequestration progresses rapidly. It may manifest with left upper quadrant pain and splenomegaly and can progress to shock. These patients are critically ill.
       c. Abdominal pain is not a reliable indicator. Bedside ultrasound may be useful in assessing for splenomegaly by measuring size.[10]
       d. This sequestration is more common in children.
     - Hemolysis: Hemolytic crisis will cause an elevation in lactate dehydrogenase, aspartate aminotransaminase/alanine aminotransferase, and bilirubin. This elevation will differentiate it from splenic sequestration.[2]
2. There is no acute anemia.
   - There are cardiopulmonary symptoms.
     - Acute chest syndrome
       a. Diagnostic criteria are any combination of fever, shortness of breath, hypoxia, and/or chest pain with new infiltrate on CXR.[11,12]
       b. Multifactorial cause (**Box 1**)
   - Absence of cardiopulmonary symptoms
     - Vasoocclusive crisis[14]: This condition causes ischemic pain.

Box 1
Possible causes of acute chest syndrome

- Acute chest syndrome is often the result of pulmonary microvascular emboli, fat emboli, and/or infection.
- Resulting hypoxia and respiratory splinting worsen hypoxemia.[13]
- Hypoxemia increases sickling, thus, worsening vasoocclusion, worsening symptoms.
- Ischemia causes free radical formation and upregulation of vascular endothelial adhesive molecules, worsening vasoocclusion.[1]
- Pulmonary infections often precipitate or are comorbid with acute chest syndrome.

1. Bones, joints, and muscles are commonly affected.
2. Rarely, it can cause myonecrosis.[15]
3. Creatine phosphokinase may be used in the appropriate setting.
4. Ensure patients are not developing osteomyelitis, septic arthritis, avascular necrosis, or another emergent cause. Ask patients if their pain is similar or different than usual.

o Infarction: Patients are at a higher risk for infarction because of sickling of cells. Providers must have an increased suspicion of embolic disease in patients with SCD, as they are at higher risk for it, despite age or other risk factors.[7,16]
1. Stroke
2. Pulmonary thrombosis or pulmonary embolism
3. Venous thromboembolism
4. Renal infarction
5. Priapism
6. Splenic infarction
7. Chronic microvascular infarctions (often reduce or eliminate splenic function reducing immune function)
8. Hepatic infarction (may be difficult to differentiate from hepatitis or biliary disease)

Treatment

1. Aplastic crisis[2]
   - Bone marrow suppression is often self-limited, but patients with SCD may not be able to tolerate an acute drop in RBC production.
   - PRBC transfusion is indicated if HgB drops more than 2 g/dL from baseline.
   - This condition is usually self-limited and resolves in 1 week.
2. Splenic sequestration
   - Initially, fluid resuscitate if patients are in shock to bridge to transfusion, as fluids may help the spleen release sequestered RBCs.
   - Perform a packed RBC (PRBC) transfusion to goal Hgb of 6 to 8 g/dL.[17]
   - Rule out precipitating pathology, such as infection.
   - Splenectomy is not routinely indicated.
3. Hemolysis
   - This condition is often self-limited.
   - PRBC should be performed if transfusion is required, though often it is not.[1]
   - Rule out precipitating pathology.
4. Acute chest syndrome
   - Aggressive pain treatment can be required to reduce splinting and increase tidal volume. This treatment will lead to improved respiratory mechanics and help improve oxygenation, potentially helping reduce sickling.[11]
   - Opioids are the preferred method of pain control. Although aggressive treatment is recommended, caution must be used to avoid oversedation causing hypoventilation.
     o Antiinflammatories may be used, though with caution. Patients with SCD have microvascular renal disease, even in the setting of normal creatinine due to chronic renal vasculopathy from SCD.[18]
   - Begin incentive spirometry on admission. It reduces splinting, increases tidal volume, and is an affective adjunct to pain medications in the treatment of acute chest syndrome.[19]
   - Bronchodilators are indicated if wheezing is present.[20]
   - Supplemental oxygen is recommended only if patients are hypoxic.

- Administer antibiotics to cover for infection. Typically a macrolide plus third-generation cephalosporin are used.[7] There is not, however, clear evidence for a specific antibiotic choice.[21]
- Perform parenteral hydration. The goal of hydration in the treatment of ACS, or really any SCD complication, is to decrease plasma viscosity. Hypotonic solutions are preferred.[2,22]
- Hydration is only indicated for patients with hypovolemia or examination findings suggesting dehydration.
- Hypotonic solutions create an osmotic gradient that allows fluid to be taken up by the RBCs, rehydrating the RBCs and reducing sickling.
- D5 1/4 normal saline should be given at 1.0 to 1.5 times the maintenance rate.
- Avoid normal saline bolus, as it may precipitate acute chest syndrome. Normal saline, or any normotonic/hypertonic IV fluid, can have the opposite effect, drawing fluids out of RBCs and worsening sickling, which may worsen acute chest syndrome.[7]
- Perform exchange transfusion.[7,23]
  - This transfusion method removes sickled cells while maintaining blood viscosity. Removing sickled cells reduces microvascular occlusion, whereas the transfusion of normal cells improves oxygen carrying capacity and reduces tissue hypoxia. It is thought to be lifesaving, but there is limited evidence on its efficacy (**Box 2**).
5. Vasoocclusion
- Pain crisis: As mentioned earlier, pain crisis is a common reason for a visit to the ED; patients are generally on outpatient pain medications and have written plans for treating pain exacerbations. Many patients may have developed a tolerance to opioids because of routine use and will require more aggressive treatment.
  - Opioid medications are preferred.[2]
    1. Morphine 0.1 mg/kg every 15 to 30 minutes
    2. Hydromorphone 0.015 mg/kg every 15 to 30 minutes
  - Intranasal fentanyl 2 mcg/kg may be a useful adjunct, especially in children.[24]
  - Ketamine 0.3 mg/kg may be a useful adjunct in opioid-tolerant patients.[17]
  - Use caution with antiinflammatory drugs because of underlying renal dysfunction.
  - Many patients know dosing regimens that work for them. Because of this, their requests for specific medications can be interpreted as drug seeking. Evidence has borne out that although some patients with SCD may be seeking opiates for elicit purposes, most are not.[25]
  - Supplemental oxygen and hydration are often not necessary.
    - Supplemental oxygen is only needed if patients are hypoxic.[7]
    - IV hydration is not routinely needed. If indicated, oral hydration is preferred. Gentle IV hydration can be used if indicated. Avoid boluses if possible.

Box 2
Indications for exchange transfusion

- Extremis with a Pao_2 level less than 60 mm Hg is an indication. This treatment seems to be more effective for patients with higher HgB levels (>9 mg/dL).
- It may also be considered in the treatment of stroke, priapism, or other life-threatening vasoocclusive conditions.

- Ensure pain (ie, chest pain, abdominal pain, headache) is not a result of another pathologic process.
- Embolic disease
  - Patients are at much higher risk for embolic diseases, such as stroke, pulmonary embolism, and renal/splenic/hepatic infarction. Have a high index of suspicion when patients with SCD present with signs and symptoms concerning for any of these embolic pathology despite their age or lack of other risk factors.
  - Treatment depends on the type of infarction and often involves routine care indicated for the specific condition; however, gentle hydration and exchange transfusion may be useful adjuncts in these cases as well.

CASE SUMMARY

The patient presented with concerns for a possible flulike illness. After the workup, he was found to have acute chest syndrome based on his constellation of symptoms and presence of new infiltrate on CXR. He was admitted for further therapy. He was found to be hypoxemic on his initial ABG. Exchange transfusion was started with improvement of symptoms. He had a prolonged course in the hospital, but with aggressive pain control and incentive spirometry he had greatly improved respiratory mechanics. The antibiotic course was completed despite the blood and sputum cultures being negative. He was discharged home with hematology follow-up.

CASE DISCUSSION

Patients with SCD have a disease that puts them at risk for multiple comorbid conditions, many of which are severe. SCD predisposes them to have recurrent ED visits. This circumstance can cause cognitive bias of providers against these patients putting patients and providers at risk of bad outcomes. Care must be taken to be aware of this when evaluating patients with SCD. SCD is a painful, life-long disease and deserves to be treated appropriately. Lack of pain control can cause a worsening of the condition, such as respiratory splinting, which can cause hypoxemia and increased sickling. This result may precipitate acute chest syndrome or other SCD-related conditions.

It is often difficult to differentiate symptoms of another pathology, whether minor or severe, from sickle cell–related symptoms. Have a strong suspicion for possible sickle cell–related illness masked by misleading complaints, as in the aforementioned example whereby the patient's concerns were for influenza, which was then diagnosed as the life-threatening acute chest syndrome. Patients may know their usual pain, and it is useful to ask them if they think their symptoms are typical of their SCD pain or if it seems different. They may know other useful information, such as their baseline HbG. Taking a good history is critical in managing patients with SCD.

The life span of patients with SCD has increased greatly over the last few years. This increase is in large part due to early detection of the disease and improved preventative care. Emergency providers play a critical role in early detection and treatment of life-threatening sickle cell–related complications. Having a good understanding of these and a diagnostic plan aids in efficient detection and treatment.

Sickle cell crises are intensely painful. Expert guidelines recommend aggressive pain control. This control includes repeated dosing of opiates at frequent intervals. Some of these patients may require more frequent use of the ED for adequate pain control. Be sure to treat patients appropriately, understanding their pain-control regimens will often require more frequent dosing of medications than providers may be used to administering.

Pattern recognition

- Check for acute anemia, defined as an Hgb drop of 2 mg/dL from patients' baseline.
- If anemic, the next step is to check the reticulocyte count to differentiate hemolysis/sequestration from aplastic crisis.
- If there is no significant anemia, assess for cardiopulmonary symptoms. Conduct a workup for acute chest syndrome if present.
- Differentiate pain crises from other mimicking pathology.

REFERENCES

1. Tintinalli JE. Emergency medicine: a comprehensive study guide. New York: McGraw-Hill; 2011.
2. Raam R, Mallemat H, Jhun P, et al. Sickle cell crisis and you: a how-to guide. Ann Emerg Med 2016;67(6):787–90.
3. Paul RN, Castro OL, Aggarwal A, et al. Acute chest syndrome: sickle cell disease. Eur J Haematol 2011;87(3):191–207.
4. Bender MA. Sickle cell disease. GeneReviews® [Internet]. Seattle (WA): University of Washington, Seattle; 2003. p. 1993–2017 [updated August 17, 2017].
5. Damy T, Bodez D, Habibi A, et al. Haematological determinants of cardiac involvement in adults with sickle cell disease. Eur Heart J 2015;37(14):1158–67.
6. Cochrane. Inhaled drugs for opening up the airways in cases of acute chest syndrome in people with sickle cell disease | Cochrane. Available at: http://www.cochrane.org/CD003733/CF_inhaled-drugs-opening-airways-cases-acute-chest-syndrome-people-sickle-cell-disease. Accessed November 9, 2017.
7. Available at: http://www.nhlbi.nih.gov/health-pro/guidelines/sickle-cell-disease-guidelines. (Evidence-based management of sickle cell disease: expert panel report, 2014). Accessed October 15, 2017.
8. dos Santos Brito Silva Furtado M, Viana MB, Rrios JSH, et al. Prevalence and incidence of erythrovirus B19 infection in children with sickle cell disease: the impact of viral infection in acute clinical events. J Med Virol 2015;88(4):588–95.
9. Naymagon L, Pendurti G, Billett HH. Acute splenic sequestration crisis in adult sickle cell disease: a report of 16 cases. Hemoglobin 2015;39(6):375–9.
10. Lee M, Roberts JM, Chen L, et al. Estimation of spleen size with hand-carried ultrasound. J Ultrasound Med 2014;33(7):1225–30.
11. Wright J. Acute chest syndrome in sickle cell disease. In: Practical management of haemoglobinopathies. p. 88–98. https://doi.org/10.1002/9780470988398.ch10.
12. Allareddy V, Roy A, Lee MK, et al. Outcomes of acute chest syndrome in adult patients with sickle cell disease: predictors of mortality. PLoS One 2014;9(4). https://doi.org/10.1371/journal.pone.0094387 [exchange transfusion].
13. Salzman SH. Does splinting from thoracic bone ischemia and infarction contribute to the acute chest syndrome in sickle cell disease? Chest 2002;122(1):6–9.
14. Lovett PB, Sule HP, Lopez BL. Sickle cell disease in the emergency department. Hematol Oncol Clin North Am 2017;31(6):1061–79.
15. Tageja N, Racovan M, Valent J, et al. Myonecrosis in sickle cell anemia—overlooked and underdiagnosed. Case Rep Med 2010;2010:1–3.
16. Novelli EM. Gladwin MT2 crises in sickle cell disease. Chest 2016;149(4):1082–93.

17. Sin B, Tatunchak T, Paryavi M, et al. The use of ketamine for acute treatment of pain: a randomized, double-blind, placebo-controlled. J Emerg Med 2017;52(5):601.
18. Al-Salem A. Renal complications of sickle cell anemia. Med Surg Complications Sickle Cell Anemia 2015;271–80.
19. Incentive spirometry to prevent acute pulmonary complications in sickle cell diseases. J Pediatr 1996;128(3):434–5. https://doi.org/10.1016/s0022-3476(96)70298-6.
20. Knight-Madden JM, Hambleton IR. Inhaled bronchodilators for acute chest syndrome in people with sickle cell disease. Cochrane Database Syst Rev 2016;(9):CD003733.
21. Dastgiri S, Dolatkhah R. Blood transfusions for treating acute chest syndrome in people with sickle cell disease. Cochrane Database Syst Rev 2016:CD007843. https://doi.org/10.1002/14651858.cd007843.pub3.
22. McGann PT, Nero AC, Ware RE. Current management of sickle cell anemia. Cold Spring Harb Perspect Med 2013;3(8):a011817.
23. Cheung AT, Miller JW, Miguelino MG, et al. Exchange transfusion therapy and its effects on real-time microcirculation in pediatric sickle cell anemia patients. J Pediatr Hematol Oncol 2012;34(3):169–74.
24. Fein DM, Avner JR, Scharbach K, et al. Intranasal fentanyl for initial treatment of vaso-occlusive crisis in sickle cell disease. Pediatr Blood Cancer 2017;64(6). https://doi.org/10.1002/pbc.26332.
25. Udezue E, Herrera E, Herrera E. Pain management in adult acute sickle cell pain crisis: a view point. West Afr J Med 2008;26(3). https://doi.org/10.4314/wajm.v26i3.28305.

Rapid Fire: Superior Vena Cava Syndrome

Shelly Zimmerman, DO[a,b,]*, Matthew Davis, DO[a,1]

KEYWORDS

- Superior vena cava syndrome (SVCS) • Thrombosis • CT scan • Radiotherapy
- Chemotherapy • Stenting • Carcinoma • Non-Hodgkin lymphoma

KEY POINTS

- Superior vena cava syndrome (SVCS) occurs when there is mechanical obstruction of the superior vena cava caused by either external compression, neoplastic invasion of the vessel wall, or internal obstruction.
- The most common cause of SVCS is malignancy. Small cell lung cancer and non-Hodgkin lymphoma are the most common culprits, though intravascular devices with associated thrombosis are becoming a more common cause.
- Classic symptoms and findings in SVCS include edema of the face, neck, and upper extremity; shortness of breath and cough; plethora of the face and neck; distended veins in the neck and chest; and head ache and hoarseness.
- The treatment of SVCS in the emergency department is mostly supportive, with head elevation, oxygen, and steroids; emergent intervention is rarely required.
- Definitive treatment of SVCS typically includes both radiotherapy and chemotherapy, and, intravascular therapy with stenting is increasingly considered.

Case: superior vena cava syndrome (SCVS) associated with lung malignancy.

Pertinent History: A 65-year-old man presents to the emergency department (ED) via emergency medical services with a complaint of shortness of breath. The patient has a history of lung cancer. The patient's tumor was first discovered 2 months prior and needle biopsy was performed that revealed squamous cell carcinoma. PET scans revealed metastatic disease. The patient stated that he awoke at 6 AM and began feeling progressively short of breath. The patient complained of productive cough with a large amount of sputum, which resulted in the shortness

Disclosure Statement: The authors have no conflict of interest.
[a] Emergency Medicine Residency, Norman Regional Health Systems, GME Office, 901 North Porter, Norman, OK 73071, USA; [b] Department of Family Medicine, Oklahoma State University College of Osteopathic Medicine, 1111 West 17th Street, # A247, Tulsa, OK 74107, USA
[1] Present address: 11708 Milano Road, Oklahoma City, OK 73173.
* Corresponding author. Norman Regional Health Systems, GME Office, 901 North Porter, Norman, OK 73071.
E-mail address: szimmerman@nrh-ok.com

Emerg Med Clin N Am 36 (2018) 577–584
https://doi.org/10.1016/j.emc.2018.04.011
0733-8627/18/© 2018 Elsevier Inc. All rights reserved.

emed.theclinics.com

of breath. He also complained of hoarseness and difficulty speaking with right-sided neck swelling that had been present for some time and seemed to be worsening. The patient denied fever, chills, headache, chest pain, wheezing, abdominal pain, nausea, or vomiting. He had a previous episode of shortness of breath 3 days before, was seen in the ED, placed on levofloxacin, and was discharged home. The patient had received several radiation treatments but no chemotherapy.

Social History: former smoker, no drug or alcohol use.

Past Medical History: lung cancer, chronic obstructive pulmonary disease.

Medications: aspirin Enteric Coated, Esomeprazole, magnesium oxide, metoprolol, fish oil, oxycodone, Umeclidinium bromide and vilanterol, diphenhydramine, prednisone

Pertinent Physical Examination: Temperature: 36.4°C, blood pressure: 150/88, heart rate: 118, Respiratory Rate: 26, Oxygen Saturation: 87% on room air.

General: alert with no immediate need for airway protection or signs of toxicity. The patient does appear to be mildly short of breath.

Ear, Nose and Throat: the patient has a notably hoarse voice.

• Eyes: pupils equal and round, no pallor or injection.
• Face: flushed and edematous.
• Mouth: mucous membranes are moist.

Neck: neck is supple, nontender. Jugular Venous Distension present. Right neck swelling. Neck is flushed.

Respiratory: wheezing bilaterally in all lung fields with decreased breath sounds at the right lower base.

Cardiovascular: tachycardia with regular rhythm.

Gastrointestinal: abdomen is soft and nontender, no masses, bowel sounds are normal.

Neurologic: no altered mental status or confusion. No focal deficits appreciated.

Skin: warm and dry. dilation of upper extremity veins.

Musculoskeletal: mild pitting edema in the bilateral lower extremities. Extremities are nontender with full range of motion.

Diagnostic testing	
	0740
White blood cell count	$7.2*10^9$/L
Hemoglobin	11.7 G/DL
Sodium	128 mmol/L
pH	7.431 mmol/L
Lactate	7.53 mmoL/L
Creatinine	0.78 mG/DL
Glucose	299 mG/DL

Computed tomography (CT) chest Pulmonary Embolus protocol: no pulmonary emboli, new right middle lobe pneumonia, multiple masses right lung again noted compatible with patient's history of known malignancy. Mass effect on the superior vena cava (SVC).

Clinical Course: Sputum cultures from prior visit 3 days before grew out *Pseudomonas* sensitive to ciprofloxacin. Cultures were not sensitive to levofloxacin. The patient's oncologist was contacted, who thought the patient required admission to the care of the hospitalist with a cardiology consult for possible urgent SVC stent placement. The patient's immediate symptoms of productive cough, shortness of breath, and room air hypoxia were thought to be secondary to both pneumonia and SVCS. The patient was started on ciprofloxacin. The patient's oxygen saturations responded well to oxygen by nasal cannula at 5 L. The patient was admitted to the care of the hospitalist with consults to the oncologist and cardiologist.

LEARNING POINTS
Introduction or Background

SVCS occurs when there is mechanical obstruction of the SVC caused by either external compression, neoplastic invasion of vessel wall, or internal obstruction. It was first described by Hunter[1] in 1757 in a patient with a large syphilitic aneurysm. With the use of antibiotics, the role of infections in SVCS has declined while malignancy has become the most common culprit, with lung cancer and non-Hodgkin lymphoma at the top of the differential list.[2-4] Not to be ignored is an increasing incidence of SVCS caused by a benign cause. Various intravascular devices with associated thrombosis are commonly placed in oncology patients.[2,4,5]

Physiology or Pathophysiology

1. The SVC is a thin-walled, low-pressure vein that provides the route for most of the blood that drains back to the heart from the head, neck, upper extremities, and upper thorax. In its location in the right mediastinum, it can be easily compressed by abnormalities in associated structures such as the trachea, right bronchus, aorta, pulmonary artery, or perihilar and paratracheal lymph nodes. Impairment of blood flow through the SVC leads to venous engorgement proximal to the site of the obstruction, resulting in the classic signs and symptoms.[6] Collateral blood flow into the azygous venous system or inferior vena cava then occurs with dilation of these collateral systems over time.[7]

2. Approximately 90% of all cases of SVCS are the result of malignancy, with 75% of the malignant cases secondary to lung cancer and 15% secondary to non-Hodgkin lymphoma.[4,5,8-10] Breast cancer, esophageal cancer, germ cell tumors, thymoma, thyroid carcinoma, and metastatic disease make up the remaining malignant causes.[5,8,11,12] Right-sided lung cancer is more likely to cause SVCS,[5,13] with small cell lung cancer being the most common type.[2] SVCS is more common in men because lung cancer is more common in men and this syndrome presents most commonly in patients at the age of 50 years or older.[6]

3. Benign causes for SVCS should also be considered in patients presenting with concerning symptoms. These include intravascular devices with associated thrombosis, cardiac causes, mediastinal fibrosis, benign mediastinal tumors, vascular disease, and infections.[4,5,11,14]

Making the Diagnosis

A high index of suspicion for both a patient at risk for cancer and for the symptoms and signs of SVCS is required to make the diagnosis.

1. History: The patient presenting to the ED with SVCS will most likely present with complaints of shortness of breath. Dyspnea occurs in 63% of these patients.[6,15] Dyspnea, as well as cough, is more likely to occur in patients presenting with SVCS associated with a malignancy versus a benign cause.[3,16] Other symptoms can include facial, neck, and arm swelling; headache, lightheadedness, or head fullness; distorted vision; nasal stuffiness; hoarseness; stridor; chest pain;

dysphagia; and nausea.[7,15] Symptoms can present very acutely or can come on over months. This depends on the rapidity of the SVC obstruction. The more acute it is in onset, the more severe the symptoms will be to the patient owing to the lack of time for development and enlargement of the collateral venous systems.[17,18]

2. Physical: The most common physical examination finding is facial and neck edema. Distended neck and chest veins are also commonly seen.[2,3,16] Extremity swelling, plethora, alterations in mental status, and papilledema can be present. Laryngeal, bronchial, and cerebral edema are rare but potentially deadly findings that can be associated with the increased intravenous (IV) pressures associated with SVCS.[17,19]

Summary of presenting features

- Consider SVCS in a patient with a known diagnosis of lung cancer or non-Hodgkin lymphoma or risk factors for these diseases or in patients with indwelling devices in their SVC.
- Patients will present with complaints that can include
  - Shortness of breath
  - Cough
  - Headache (often worse with lying flat or bending over)
  - Facial, neck, and or arm swelling or edema (often worse in the morning)
  - Hoarseness
  - Distended neck and chest wall veins

---

3. Diagnostic evaluation
   - Chest radiograph may provide limited information in cases in which SVCS is suspected. It can reveal evidence of mass, perihilar lymphadenopathy, and mediastinal disease.
   - Venography, once thought to be the gold standard for diagnosis, can provide information about the exact location of obstruction, though it is not performed frequently in the ED.
   - CT scanning with IV contrast provides the emergency physician with not only the diagnosis of SVCS but also important diagnostic information about the cause, which can guide treatment. A CT scan can determine whether there is external compression, thrombus, or both. If caused by malignancy, it can provide diagnostic and staging information about the malignancy.[20] The sensitivity and specificity for CT scanning is 96% and 92%, respectively.[16,21] **Fig. 1** demonstrates the superiority of CT scan compared with chest radiograph by placing images from the same patient next to each other.
   - Ultrasound, both bedside and formal, can provide information about the presence and extent of thrombus and can point to obstruction. Though the SVC cannot be directly visualized with ultrasound, the venous waveform in the subclavian and brachiocephalic veins may show dampening and loss of venous pulsatility, and minimal respiratory variation, when the SVC is obstructed.[22]
   - MRI may be useful in the ED setting when patients are allergic to IV contrast or have renal failure.[23]

Treatment

Urgency or emergency?

Once thought to be an oncologic emergency, SVCS syndrome rarely requires emergent treatment in the ED or arrangement for emergent radiotherapy or stenting.[24,25]

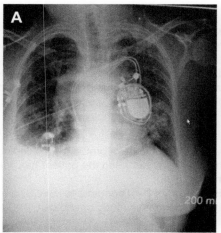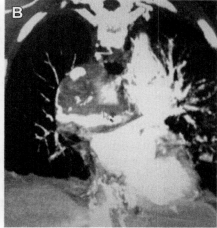

Fig. 1. (A) Chest radiograph of a patient with upper mediastinal mass. Contrasted chest CT of the same patient in (B) more clearly demonstrates the mediastinal mass as well as SVCS. (*Courtesy of* C. Kaide, MD, Wexner Medical Center at The Ohio State University.)

Rarely, it can cause significant airway obstruction secondary to laryngeal edema or cerebral edema. SVCS is most often an urgency and patients need to be directed toward appropriate care. If the patient is stable, a histologic diagnosis should be established first.[26] In the ED, improvement in symptoms can be obtained with supplemental oxygen, elevation of the head of the bed, and a course of parental steroids.[4,5] Initiating anticoagulant therapy or giving thrombolytic therapy in the ED should be considered when associated thrombus is noted.

1. Radiation and chemotherapy: radiation therapy is a mainstay of treatment in SVCS secondary to non-small cell carcinomas of the lung.[6] Shrinking the size of the tumor often provides relief of the obstruction. Chemotherapy should also be considered in patients with chemosensitive tumors.[27]
2. Endovascular therapy: endovascular therapy can be beneficial in the treatment of SVCS and can include stenting, percutaneous transluminal angioplasty, and intravascular thrombolysis.[28] There is mounting evidence that these procedures may be the best treatment in SVSC of benign origin.[29] In malignant SVCS, stents can be used to relieve symptoms while the histologic diagnosis is being perused.[30] If chemotherapy and radiotherapy have failed, stenting is recommended.[31–33] There is also mounting evidence that stenting should be the first-line consideration in patients with malignancy associated SVCS secondary to the superior rate of symptom improvement and higher rate of response to treatment.[17,34] Associated short-term anticoagulation needed with stent placement may preclude the placement if surgical procedures are planned.[18]

DISPOSITION

Consider admitting patients requiring anticoagulation or thrombolysis, those with new cancer diagnosis, and those with moderate to severe symptoms.[34] Patients with mild symptoms and in the care of an oncologist can be referred for outpatient evaluation and treatment.

CASE CONCLUSION

After admission to the hospital, the patient was successfully stented by cardiology. After stenting, the patient's symptoms progressively worsened, despite care. The patient became increasingly hoarse and developed esophageal dysphagia secondary to tumor compression from the extensive disease. He began to require high-flow oxygen and became more anemic. After speaking with the family and patient, comfort measures were instituted and the patient died 2 days later.

CASE DISCUSSION

1. As noted in this case, SVCS can present among a multitude of problems so keeping a high index of suspicion and considering the diagnosis when the patient has risk factors for this disease process is imperative.
2. A careful history and physical examination will often be diagnostic for SVCS.
3. In the ED, CT scanning with IV contrast is the diagnostic study of choice.

Pattern recognition

SVCS

- Upper body plethora (often positional)
- Headache (often positional)
- Dyspnea
- History suspicious for cancer
- History of indwelling catheters or pacemaker leads

REFERENCES

1. Hunter W. The history of an aneurysm of the aorta, with some remarks on aneurysms in general. London: Med Obs Inq; 1757. p. 323–57.
2. Ahmann FR. A reassessment of the clinical implications of superior vena caval syndrome. J Clin Oncol 1984;2:961–9.
3. Wilson LD, Detterbeck FC, Yahalom J. Clinical practice: Superior vena cava syndrome with malignant causes. N Engl J Med 2007;356:1862–9.
4. Cheng S. Superior vena cava syndrome: a contemporary review of a historic disease. Cardiol Rev 2009;17:16–23.
5. Ostler PJ, Clark DP, Watkinson AF, et al. Superior vena cava obstruction: a modern management strategy. Clin Oncol (R Coll Radiol) 1997;9:83–9.
6. Armstrong BA, Perez CA, Simpson JR, et al. Role of irradiation in the management of superior vena cava syndrome. Int J Radiat Oncol Biol Phys 1987;4:531–9.
7. Kim HJ, Kim HS, Chung SH. CT diagnosis of superior vena cava syndrome: importance of collateral vessels. AJR Am J Roentgenol 1993;161:539–42.
8. Lochridge SK, Knibbe WP, Doty DB. Obstruction of the superior vena cava. Surgery 1979;85:14–24.
9. Nogeire C, Mincer F, Botstein C. Long survival in patients with bronchogenic carcinoma complicated by superior vena cava obstruction. Chest 1979;75:325–9.
10. Perez-Soler R, McLaughlin P, Velaquez WS, et al. Clinical features and results of management of superior vena cava syndrome secondary to lymphoma. J Clin Oncol 1984;2:260–6.

11. Nieto AF, Doty DB. Superior vena cava obstruction: clinical syndrome, etiology and treatment. Curr Probl Cancer 1986;10(9):441–84.
12. Bigsby R, Greengrass R, Unruh H. Diagnostic algorithm for acute superior vena caval obstruction (SVCO). J Cardiovasc Surg (Torino) 1993;4:347–50.
13. Houman M, Ksontini I, Ghorbell Ben, et al. Association of right heart thrombosis, endomyocardial fibrosis, and pulmonary artery aneurysm in Bechet's disease. EUR J Intern Med 2002;7:455.
14. Parish JM, Marschke RF Jr, Dines DE. Etiological considerations in superior vena cava syndrome. Mayo Clin Proc 1981;7:407–13.
15. Rice TW, Rodriguez RM, Light RW. The superior vena cava syndrome: clinical characteristics and evolving etiology. Medicine (Baltimore) 2006;85(1):37–42.
16. Kahn UA, Shanholtz CB, McCurdy MT. Oncologic mechanical emergencies. Emerg Med Clin North Am 2014;32(3):495–508.
17. Talapatra K, Panda S, Goyle S, et al. Superior vena cava syndrome: a radiation oncologist's perspective. J Cancer Res Ther 2016;12:515–9.
18. Wan JF, Bezjak A. Superior vena cava syndrome. Emerg Med Clin North Am 2009;27:243–55.
19. Nickloes T, Long CL, Mack LO, et al. Superior vena cava syndrome clinical presentation. Medscape. 2016. Available at: http://emedicine.medscape.com/article460865-clinical. Accessed April 22, 2017.
20. Nickloes T, Long CL, Mack LO, et al. Superior vena cava syndrome workup. Medscape. Available at: http://emedicine.medscape.com/article460865-workup. Accessed April 22, 2017.
21. Eren S, Karaman A, Okur A. The superior vena cava syndrome caused by malignant disease: imaging with multi-detector row CT. Eur J Radiol 2006;59:93–103.
22. Lv FQ, Duan YY, Yuan LJ, et al. Doppler superior vena cava flow evolution and respiratory variation in superior vena cava syndrome. Echocardiography 2008; 25(4):360–5.
23. Thornton MJ, Ryan R, Varghese JC, et al. A three-dimensional gadolinium-enhanced MR venography technique for imaging central veins. Am J Roentgenol 1999;173:999–1003.
24. Gauden SJ. Superior vena cava syndrome induced by bronchogenic carcinoma: is this an oncologic emergency? Australas Radiol 1993;38:363–6.
25. Schraufnagel DE, Hill R, Leech JA, et al. Superior vena cava obstruction. Is it a medical emergency? Am J Med 1981;70:1169–74.
26. Kvale PA, Selecky PA, Prakash UB, The American College of Chest Physicians. Palliative care in lung cancer: ACCP evidence-based clinical practice guidelines (2nd edition). Chest 2007;132:368S–403S.
27. Urban T, Lebeau B, Chastang C, et al. Superior vena cava syndrome in small-cell lung cancer. Arch Intern Med 1993;153(3):384–7.
28. Rachapalli V, Boucher LM. Superior vena cava syndrome: role of the interventionalist. Can Assoc Radiol J 2014;65(2):168–76.
29. Breault S, Doenz F, Jouannic AM, et al. Percutaneous endovascular management of chronic superior vena cava syndrome of benign causes: long term follow-up. Eur Radiol 2017;1:97–104.
30. Marcy PY, Magné N, Bentolola F, et al. Superior vena cava obstruction: is stenting necessary? Support Care Cancer 2001;9:103–7.
31. Smayra T, Otal P, Chabbert V, et al. Long-term results of endovascular stent placement in the superior vena caval system. Cardiovasc Intervent Radiol 2001;24: 388–94.

32. Thony F, Moro D, Whitmeyer P, et al. Endovascular treatment of superior vena cava obstruction in patients with malignancies. Eur Radiol 1999;9:965–71.

33. Rowell NP, Gleeson FV. Steroids, radiotherapy, chemotherapy and stents for superior vena cava syndrome in carcinoma of the bronchus. Cochrane Database Syst Rev 2001;(2):CD001316.

34. Nickloes T, Long CL, Mack LO, et al. Superior vena cava syndrome treatment and management. Medscape. 2016. Available at: http://emedicine.medscape.com/article460865-treatment. Accessed April 22, 2017.

Anticoagulation Reversal

Erica M. Simon, DO, MHA[a],*, Matthew J. Streitz, MD[a],
Daniel J. Sessions, MD[a,b], Colin G. Kaide, MD[c]

KEYWORDS

- Anticoagulant reversal • Novel oral anticoagulants • Warfarin • Heparin
- Prothrombin complex concentrate • Idarucizumab

KEY POINTS

- Four-factor prothrombin complex concentrate was designed specifically for the reversal of warfarin-associated coagulopathies.
- Reversal of heparin's anticoagulant effect may be achieved through the administration of protamine sulfate.
- Idaricuzimab is the Food and Drug Administration–approved agent for the reversal of the direct thrombin inhibitor, dabigatran.
- The use of 4-factor prothrombin complex concentrate is recommended by the American College of Cardiology and the Hemostasis and Thrombosis for the reversal of factor Xa inhibitor anticoagulation. Andexanet alfa may be considered for use in patients experiencing life-threatening or uncontrolled bleeding secondary to rivaroxaban and apixaban. Trials of the factor Xa reversal agent, aripazine are underway.
- Current guidelines for the reversal of antiplatelet therapy are lacking.

INTRODUCTION

In the United States, anticoagulant therapy is indicated for the prophylaxis and treatment of thromboembolic disorders.[1] Today, vitamin K antagonists, heparin, low-molecular-weight heparins, direct thrombin inhibitors (DTIs), and factor Xa inhibitors, are commonly used. With nearly 30 million prescriptions for warfarin written annually,[1] and more than 2.3 million individuals taking novel oral anticoagulants,[2] the clinician must be equipped with a strategy to address the most common complication of these therapies: bleeding.

THE CLOTTING CASCADE

The reversal of anticoagulation requires an understanding of the clotting cascade, a complex physiologic process used to maintain homeostasis between clot formation and degradation. In the setting of vascular endothelial injury, clot formation begins

[a] Emergency Medicine, San Antonio Uniformed Services Health Education Consortium, 3551 Roger Brooke Dr. Fort Sam, Houston, TX 78234, USA; [b] South Texas Poison Center, 7979 Wurzbach Road, San Antonio, TX 78229, USA; [c] Emergency Medicine Residency, Wexner Medical Center, The Ohio State University, 410 W. 10th Avenue, Columbus, OH, 43210, USA
* Corresponding author.
E-mail address: emsimon85@gmail.com

Emerg Med Clin N Am 36 (2018) 585–601
https://doi.org/10.1016/j.emc.2018.04.014
0733-8627/18/© 2018 Elsevier Inc. All rights reserved.

emed.theclinics.com

with primary hemostasis. During primary hemostasis, platelets bind damaged endothelium via an interaction between a glycoprotein (GP IIbIIIa) and von Willebrand factor.[3] Through platelet activation and degranulation, additional platelets are recruited to the site of injury, thereby forming a platelet plug.[3] The efficacy of the platelet plug in achieving hemostasis is a function of platelet quantity and quality. These platelet characteristics may vary according to patient comorbidities (bleeding diathesis, advanced renal disease, etc) and pharmaceutical therapy (eg, nonsteroidal antiinflammatory drugs or aspirin).[3,4]

After primary hemostasis, secondary hemostasis begins with activation of the clotting cascade. During secondary hemostasis, activated factor Xa catalyzes the conversion of prothrombin to thrombin (factor IIa). Thrombin, in turn, catalyzes the conversion of fibrinogen to fibrin.[5] Ultimately, fibrin is responsible for cross-linking and strengthening the platelet plug. The process of secondary hemostasis depends on the quantity of functional clotting factors, and their successful activation.[5]

In terms of laboratory analyses, platelet function tests and platelet aggregation assays may be used to assess primary hemostasis; however, many of these studies are time consuming and poorly standardized, limiting their clinical usefulness in the emergency setting.[4] Bleeding time is no longer used clinically. The process of secondary hemostasis is measured using prothrombin time (PT), International Normalized Ratio (INR; extrinsic and common pathways; factors II, VII, X), and activated partial thromboplastin time (aPTT; intrinsic and common pathways; all factors except factor VII).[3]

REVERSAL OF WARFARIN

In the United States, warfarin (Coumadin; Bristol-Myers-Squibb, NY) is indicated for the prophylaxis and treatment of venous thromboembolism, pulmonary embolism (PE), thromboembolic complications associated with atrial fibrillation or cardiac valve replacement, and for reduction of mortality risk secondary to emboli after myocardial infarctions (MIs) and cerebrovascular accidents. Warfarin is a vitamin K antagonist, inhibiting the hepatic enzyme vitamin K epoxide reductase, thereby limiting the synthesis of factors II, VII, IX, and X, and the anticoagulant proteins C and S. Therapeutic doses of warfarin decrease the total amount of each active vitamin K–dependent clotting factor by approximately 30% to 50%.[6] As mentioned, the PT and INR are measures of the extrinsic pathway of the coagulation cascade and are, therefore, used to monitor the anticoagulant effect of warfarin.[7]

The reversal of warfarin centers on immediate and sustained therapy. Immediate reversal is attained through the employment of prothrombin complex concentrates (PCC) and fresh frozen plasma (FFP), and sustained reversal is achieved through vitamin K administration.

Prothrombin Complex Concentrates

In the United States, PCCs are available in 3- and 4-factor preparations. Bebulin (BDI Pharma, Inc, SC) or Profilnine-SD (Grifols Inc, Spain) are 3-factor concentrates that contain factors II, IX, X, and minimal amounts of factor VII.[8] The 3-factor concentrates are approved by the US Food and Drug Administration (FDA) for the treatment of bleeding events in individuals with hemophilia B (factor IX deficiency).[9,10] In 2009, Holland and colleagues[11] published data regarding the off-label use of Profilnine for the reversal of warfarin in patients with bleeding (n = 29) or at high risk for bleeding (n = 11). Three-factor PCC alone (25 international units per kilogram [IU/kg] and 50 IU/kg doses) lowered the INR to less than 3 in 50% and 43% of patients, respectively, leading the authors to conclude that 3-factor PCC does not satisfactorily decrease supratherapeutic INRs owing to the low factor VII content.[11]

In 2013, the FDA approved Kcentra (CSL Behring, King of Prussia, PA), a 4-factor PCC, for the reversal of warfarin-related coagulopathy. Kcentra contains factors II, VII, IX, and X, in addition to proteins C and S (heparin and antithrombin III are added to maintain factors in the unactivated form).[12] Kcentra is administered intravenously with dosing recommendations based on the patient's baseline INR (the initial dose recommended is 25–50 IU/kg for significant bleeds).[12]

Activated PCC (aPCC), also known as factor VIII inhibitor-bypassing activity (FEIBA), is indicated for the treatment of bleeding episodes resulting from coagulation factors VIII or IX deficiencies.[13] FEIBA contains primarily activated factor VII and smaller quantities of activated factors II, IX, and X.[13,14] In 2009, Wójcik and colleagues[15] performed a retrospective chart review of patients who received FEIBA (n = 72) or FFP (n = 69) in the setting of life-threatening hemorrhage secondary to warfarin-induced coagulopathy. In this study, the INR of patients receiving FEIBA normalized 12 times faster than those who received FFP.[14,15] Fifty-six of the 72 patients who received FEIBA (with 10 mg of intravenous [IV] vitamin K) survived.[15] FEIBA may be considered when 4-factor PCC is not available.

PCCs are contraindicated in persons with a history of anaphylaxis to PCCs or any of their components, or those with a history of disseminated intravascular coagulation, MI, and PE (increased risk of thrombosis).[10,12,13] In terms of thrombotic risk, studies demonstrate no statistically significant difference in the incidence of thromboembolic events in patients treated with 3- and 4-factor PCC versus FFP.[16,17] Of note, aPCC (FEIBA) contains a black box warning for thromboembolic events.[13] Data from the FDA's pharmacovigiliance program revealed FEIBA administration as associated with a thrombotic incidence of 8.24 per 100,000 infusions (the majority of data are from hemophiliacs).[18]

To date, Sarode and colleagues[16] have conducted the only clinical trial that directly compares 4-factor PCC (Kcentra) with FFP. In their study, 202 patients with hemorrhage secondary to vitamin K antagonists were randomized to receive either PCC (n = 48) and IV vitamin K or FFP (n = 104) and IV vitamin K.[16] Median baseline INR was 3.90 (range, 1.8–20.0) for the 4-factor PCC group and 3.60 (range, 1.9–38.9) for the FFP group.[16] Effective hemostasis was achieved in 72% of patients who received PCC and 65% of patients given FFP.[16] Rapid INR reduction was demonstrated in 62% of those treated with PCC versus 9% of those given FFP.[16] At 24 hours after the initial infusion, the INR was similar in both groups.[16] There was no difference in the incidence of thrombotic events (8% PCC; 6% FFP).[16]

In cases in which volume administration is a major concern, PCC should be considered superior to FFP.[19] As an example, each 500 IU (25 mL) vial of 4-factor PCC is equivalent to 2 U (250 mL/U) of FFP.[19] An 80 kg individual with an INR of 10 (using reversal doses of 50 IU/kg of PCC and 15 mL/kg FFP) would require 8 vials (200 mL) of PCC or 16 U (4 L) of FFP.[19]

Fresh Frozen Plasma

FFP contains all of the coagulation factors. Although it is type specific, with individuals of the AB blood type being universal donors, Rh compatibility is not required. Risks associated with transfusion of FFP include bloodborne infections and allergic reactions. The majority of resources advise the initial administration of 2 U of FFP for isolated intracranial bleeds and 4 U for extracranial bleeds (based on the generally accepted idea that one unit of FFP corrects clotting factors by 2%–3% in a 70-kg individual); however, a volume of 10 to 15 mL/kg may be required to address life-threatening hemorrhage.[20] As mentioned, the use of FFP may be less than ideal in the reversal of anticoagulation for persons suffering from atrial fibrillation, cardiac valvular disease, and ventricular dysfunction, because significant increases in intravascular volume may result in decompensated heart failure or transfusion-associated lung injury.[20] Because the INR of FFP is 1.5, it is impossible to achieve an INR of less than 1.5 after FFP administration alone.[20] The delivery of FFP is limited secondary to the product's frozen storage, requiring 15 to 20 minutes to thaw.[20]

Vitamin K

Vitamin K is an essential cofactor in the synthesis of factors II, VII, IX, and X, and proteins C and S. Vitamin K is available in both oral and IV forms. Subcutaneous and intramuscular administration are no longer recommended owing to unpredictable absorption and the potential for hematomas.[21] Time to onset after the administration of oral vitamin K is 6 to 10 hours, with peak activity occurring within 24 to 48 hours.[21–23] Patients who are actively bleeding should receive an initial dose of 5 to 10 mg of IV vitamin K, by slow infusion, over approximately 20 minutes.[21,22] Intravenous time to onset is 1 to 2 hours, with peak effect in 12 to 24 hours.[21] Anaphylactic reactions are associated with parenteral vitamin K administration, occurring after 3 of every 10,000 doses.[22] These reactions are commonly secondary to the diluent in which the vitamin K is prepared.[22] Of note, after vitamin K administration, therapeutic anticoagulation cannot be achieved for nearly 2 weeks.[22,23] This consideration is important for providers to appreciate.

Recombinant Factor VIIa

Recombinant factor VII (rFVIIa; NovoSeven, Novo Nordisk, Bagsværd, Denmark) was developed for the treatment of bleeding episodes in individuals with factor VIII deficiency (hemophilia A), factor IX (hemophilia B), and congenital factor VII deficiency.[24] The off-label use of rFVIIa in studies of nonhemophiliac trauma patients have demonstrated no benefit as compared with placebo.[25,26] Given the increased risk of thromboembolic events, the administration of rFVIIa is no longer recommended as an adjunct for the reversal of warfarin[25,26] (**Tables 1** and **2**).

REVERSAL OF HEPARIN AND LOW-MOLECULAR-WEIGHT HEPARINS

Heparin and the low-molecular-weight heparins (enoxaparin [Lovenox], Sonafi Aventis, Bridgewater Township, NJ), dalteparin (Fragmin; Pfizer, New York, NY), and fondaparinus (Arixtra; GlaxoSmithKline, Brentford, UK) are approved for the prophylaxis and treatment of DVT and PE.[27–30] In addition to these indications, enoxaparin may be used for the treatment of acute ST-segment elevation MI, and both enoxaparin and dalteparin may be used to address ischemic complications of unstable angina and non–Q-wave MIs.[28,29] Heparin and the low-molecular-weight heparins bind to antithrombin III, activating the antithrombin III complex, which inhibits factor Xa, and exhibits a variable inhibitory effect on factor IIa (thrombin).[27–30] The aPTT is used to measure the anticoagulation effects of heparin, with a range of 1.5 to 2.5 times the control considered therapeutic.[31] The chromogenic anti–factor Xa assay is the gold standard for monitoring low-molecular-weight heparin therapy.[32]

If urgent or emergent heparin reversal is required, heparin should be discontinued and protamine sulfate initiated. Protamine sulfate is a positively charged polypeptide, capable of reversing antithrombin III inhibition.[33] Protamine dosing should be calculated based on time elapsed since heparin administration, and the dose of heparin delivered.[34] If immediately after heparin administration, 1.0 to 1.5 mg of protamine

Table 1
Managing elevated INRs or bleeding in patients treated with vitamin K antagonists

Condition	Description
INR supratherapeutic but <5.0; absent significant bleeding	Lower or omit dose. Increase frequency of monitoring. Resume therapy at a lower dose if INR more than minimally supratherapeutic.
INR ≥5.0 but ≤10.0; absent significant bleeding	Omit 1–2 doses. Increase frequency of monitoring. Resume therapy when INR therapeutic. Or omit dose. Give 1.0–2.5 mg oral vitamin K. If the patient is at increased risk of bleeding, or requires more rapid reversal for a surgical procedure, give 2–4 mg oral vitamin K; the INR should decrease within 24 h. If the INR remains elevated, additional vitamin K (1–2 mg orally) may be given.
INR >10; absent significant bleeding	Hold warfarin therapy. Give 5–10 mg oral vitamin K; the INR should decrease within 24–48 h. Increase frequency of monitoring. Administer additional vitamin K if necessary. Resume therapy when INR is therapeutic.
Serious or life-threatening bleeding	Hold warfarin therapy. Give 10 mg vitamin K by slow IV infusion, in addition to 4-factor PCC or FFP. Vitamin K may be given every 12 h.

Abbreviations: FFP, fresh frozen plasma; INR, International Normalized Ratio; PCC, prothrombin complex concentrate.

Adapted from Holbrook A, Schulman S, Witt D, et al. Evidence-based management of anticoagulant therapy: antithrombotic therapy and prevention of thrombosis 9th edition: American College of Chest Physicians Evidence-Based Clinical Practice Guidelines. Chest 2012;141:e1525–845; and Thompson L, Sidley C, Kaide C. Anticoagulation in the trauma patient. Trauma Reports. ACH Media. 2017;18(1):2; with permission.

sulfate should be given for every 100 U of heparin delivered.[9,35] If 30 to 60 minutes have elapsed since the most recent dose of heparin, 0.50 to 0.75 mg per 100 U of heparin are advised, and if greater than 2 hours since the previous dose of heparin, 0.250 to 0.375 mg per 100 U of heparin should be given.[9,35]

Table 2
Reversal agents for warfarin

Agent	Dose	Notes
Vitamin K	1.25–10 mg orally or IV	Subcutaneous and intramuscular delivery not advised.
PCC (Profilnine or Kcentra[a])	Strategy 1: INR and weight-based dosing • INR 2–4: 25 IU/kg IV push • INR ≥4–6: 35 IU/kg IV push • INR >6: 50 IU/kg IV push Strategy 2: INR-based dosing • INR <5: 500 IU • INR >5: 1000 IU Strategy 3: Fixed dose • 1500 IU	INR-based dosing is most effective with Profilnine (3-factor PCC). Fixed dosing should not be used with Profilnine. Any of the strategies may be used with Kcentra (4-factor PCC).
aPCC (FEIBA)	50–100 U/kg (U/kg)[13]	Given the risk of thromboembolic events, use should be considered only when PCC is not available.

Abbreviations: aPCC, activated prothrombin complex concentrate; INR, International Normalized Ratio; PCC, prothrombin complex concentrate.

[a] Approved by the US Food and Drug Administration for warfarin-associated coagulopathy.

Protamine sulfate may be used to reverse the anticoagulation effects of the low-molecular-weight heparins, enoxaparin, and dalteparin. It is important to note, however, that protamine is only 60% effective in reversing these anticoagulants owing to its limited ability to address factor Xa inhibition.[27] Fondaparinux is not neutralized by protamine sulfate.[36] If using protamine to reverse enoxaparin or dalteparin, it is recommended that 1 mg of protamine be administered for every milligram of these low-molecular-weight heparins previously administered (1:1 ratio).[9,35] If bleeding continues, an additional 0.5 mg per 1 mg of enoxaparin or dalteparin are advised.[9,35] Total protamine dosing should not exceed 50 mg because, at this concentration, paradoxic anticoagulation may occur secondary to factor V inhibition.[9,33] Given the risk of anaphylaxis, hypotension, and bradycardia associated with protamine, infusions should not exceed 20 mg/min.[35]

Andexanet alfa (Annexa, Portola Pharmaceuticals, South San Francisco, CA), discussed elsewhere in this article, was designed in 2008 as a reversal agent for all factor Xa inhibitors.[37] Additional data are required before making recommendations regarding the use of andexanet alfa in the reversal of heparin and low-molecular-weight heparins (ANNEXA-4 clinical trial; n = 1, enoxaparin therapy).[37]

Aripazine (PER977, Ciraparantag; Perosphere, Danbury, CT) is a synthetic molecule designed as a reversal agent for DTIs, factor Xa inhibitors, and unfractionated and low-molecular-weight heparins.[38,39] Recently, Ansell and colleagues[40] demonstrated complete reversal of enoxaparin (a single subcutaneous dose of 1.5 mg/kg), measured by a reduction of whole blood clotting time, after the administration of 100 to 300 mg aripazine in 40 healthy volunteers. Further studies are currently underway. **Table 3**

Table 3
Reversal agents for heparin and low-molecular-weight heparins

Agent	Dose	Notes

Protamine for heparin	Time elapsed since heparin dose:
	  Immediate:
	    Administer 1–1.5 mg/100 U heparin
	  30–60 min:
	    Administer 0.5–0.75 mg/100 U heparin
	  >2 h:
	    0.25–0.375 mg/100 U heparin
		Doses should not exceed 50 mg at one time given the inhibition of factor V and potential for further anticoagulation.

Protamine for low-molecular-weight heparins	Dalteparin: 1 mg of protamine neutralizes 100 U of dalteparin • If bleeding persists or aPTT remains prolonged 2–4 h after protamine: consider administration of an additional protamine dose: 0.5 mg/100 U dalteparin. Enoxaparin: if <8 h since the previous dose, give 1 mg protamine per 1 mg of enoxaparin • If 8–12 h after the previous dose of enoxaparin: 0.5 mg protamine per 1 mg enoxaparin. • If ≥12 h after previous dose of enoxaparin: protamine not required. • If bleeding persists or aPTT remains prolonged: consider administration of a second dose of protamine: 0.5 mg per 1 mg enoxaparin.	Protamine is only partially effective for the reversal of low-molecular-weight heparins. Fondaparinux is not neutralized by protamine sulfate.

Abbreviation: aPCC, activated prothrombin complex concentrate.

contains a summary of the reversal agents for heparin and the low-molecular-weight heparins.

REVERSAL OF DIRECT ORAL ANTICOAGULANTS
Direct Thrombin Inhibitors

Dabigatran etexilate mesylate (Pradaxa, Boehringer Ingelheim, Ridgefield, CT) is an oral DTI indicated for the reduction of stroke and systemic embolism in nonvalvular atrial fibrillation, for the treatment of DVT and PE, and for the prophylaxis of DVT and PE in patients who have undergone hip arthroplasty.[41] After hepatic metabolism, dabigatran binds the active site of free and clot-bound thrombin, inhibiting the conversion of fibrinogen to fibrin, and the feedback activation of factors VII, XI, and V.[41–44]

Given its reliable dose-proportional pharmacokinetics, laboratory monitoring of dabigatran's anticoagulant effect is rarely performed.[41,42] INR response to DTIs is variable, and offers poor correlation to anticoagulation effect.[41,45] At therapeutic levels, dabigatran prolongs the ecarin clotting time, diluted thrombin time, and aPTT.[41] An elevated aPTT suggests at least therapeutic dabigatran effect, but a normal aPTT does not rule out dabigatran effect. A normal dilute thrombin time effectively excludes dabigatran effect.[42]

In 2015, the FDA approved idarucizumab (Praxbind, Boehringer Ingelheim), a humanized monoclonal antibody fragment, for the reversal of dabigatran in the setting of emergent/urgent surgical procedures, and life-threatening or uncontrolled bleeding.[46] The recommended dose of idarucizumab is 5 g, provided as 2 separate vials containing 2.5 g/50 mL, administered no more than 15 minutes apart (data available for recommendation regarding repeat dosing is limited).[46] Although a preexisting IV line may be used, per the manufacturer's guidelines, the line must be flushed with sterile sodium chloride before infusion, and no other infusion should be administered in parallel via the same access site.[46]

In a recent, multicenter, open-label single cohort trial (RE-VERSE AD [A Study of the RE-VERSal Effects of Idarucizumab on Active Dabigatran] clinical trial), 5 g of idarucizumab were administered to patients who received dabigatran therapy (group A [n = 301], 98 patients with intracranial hemorrhage, 137 with gastrointestinal bleeding; group B [n = 202], patients requiring an urgent surgical procedure).[47] The median maximum percentage of dabigatran reversal, as determined by diluted thrombin time or ecarin clotting time, in both groups was 100% (95% confidence interval, 100–100).[47] In group A, the median time to cessation of bleeding among patients with intracranial hemorrhage was 11.4 hours, and the median time to cessation of bleeding in patients with gastrointestinal bleeding was 3.5 hours.[47] In group B, the median time to procedure was 1.6 hours, with periprocedural hemostasis identified as normal in 188 patients.[47] Ninety days after idarucizumab administration, 19 individuals in group A and 15 in group B had experienced a thrombotic event.[47] Mortality rates were 18.8% and 18.9%, respectively.[47] It is worth mentioning that although the RE-VERSE AD clinical trial did not report results in terms of aPTT, the advised mechanism of assessing dabigatran therapy; these data are detailed in the text of the publication, where the authors note a good correlation between aPTT and the more specialized direct thrombin and ecarin clotting times.[48]

In situations where idarucizumab is not available, given the predominately renal excretion of dagibatran, hemodialysis should be performed.[49,50] The American Society of Hematology also recommends consideration of the administration of PCC or aPCC for life-threatening bleeds; however, this practice is supported by limited, poor-quality evidence, and is not without thrombotic risk.[51] (A 2012 randomized crossover, ex vivo, study in 10 healthy male volunteers assessed reversal of dabigatran and rivaroxaban with PCC, rFVIIa, and FEIBA: only FEIBA seemed to demonstrate the reversal profile of interest.[52]) For control and prevention of bleeding, 50 to 100 U/kg of aPCC or 50 U/kg of PCC are advised.[13,52] Cryoprecipitate administration (2 pools) is advised for patients with fibrinogen levels of less than 200 mg/dL.[48] **Table 4** contains a summary of reversal agents for DTIs.

Factor Xa Inhibitors

Factor Xa inhibitors include rivaroxaban (Xarelto; Janssen Pharmaceuticals, Raritan, NJ), apixaban (Eliquis; Bristol-Myers Squibb Company, Wallingford, CT), edoxaban (Savayasa; Daiichi Sankyo Inc, Basking Ridge, NJ), and betrixaban (Bevyxxa, Portola Pharmaceuticals). In the United States, the factor Xa inhibitors have been approved for the risk reduction of stroke and systemic embolism in patients with nonvalvular atrial fibrillation.[53–56] In addition, rivaroxaban is indicated for DVT and PE prophylaxis in patients undergoing hip or knee arthroplasty, edoxaban is approved for the treatment of DVT/PE after initial parenteral therapy, and betrixaban is approved for venous thromboembolism prophylaxis in hospitalized patients.[53,55,56] Rivaroxaban, apixaban, edoxaban, and betrixaban selectively block the active site of factor Xa, when free or bound to the prothrombinase complex.[53–56] By inhibiting factor Xa, these novel anticoagulants indirectly inhibit platelet aggregation induced by thrombin. Peak plasma concentrations are achieved within 2 hours of administration of rivaroxaban, apixaban, and edoxaban, and within 4 hours of betrixaban dosing.[52,53] After oral administration, in patients with normal renal function, elimination half-lives of the novel anticoagulants are less than 12 hours.[53–56]

At therapeutic doses, all factor Xa inhibitors prolong clotting time tests (PT, INR, aPTT); however, responses are variable, and are not useful in monitoring anticoagulation effects.[52,57] Inhibition of factor Xa and rivaroxaban are closely correlated.[57] Standardized kits using rivaroxaban calipers and controls are preferred, but may not be widely available.[57,58] (A normal PT/INR or normal anti–factor Xa excludes significant rivaroxaban levels).[57,58] To assess the anticoagulation effect of apixaban, anti–factor Xa activity, calibrated with apixaban controls, is recommended.[57,58] (Normal anti–factor Xa excludes significant apixaban levels).[57,58] Finally, anti–factor Xa activity, calibrated with heparin or edoxaban, is the recommended assay for an assessment of the extent of edoxaban anticoagulation.[57,58]

Andexanet alfa (Annexa; Portola Pharmaceuticals), as mentioned, was designed as a reversal agent for all factor Xa inhibitors.[37] A recombinant, modified, factor Xa

Table 4
Reversal agents for direct thrombin inhibitors

Agent	Dose	Notes
Idarucizumab	5 g, provided by the manufacturer as 2 vials containing 2.5 g/50 mL	Data regarding repeat dosing lacking.
PCC (Profilnine or Kcentra[a])	50 U/kg	
FEIBA	50–100 U/kg	
Cryoprecipitate	2 pools	Administer for patients with fibrinogen <200 mg/dL.

[a] Approved by the US Food and Drug Administration for warfarin-associated coagulopathy.
Data from Refs.[13,47,48,52]

molecule, andexanet alfa competes with native factor Xa to bind Xa inhibitors, thereby eliminating their anticoagulant effect.[37] Completed phase III clinical trials identified rapid restoration of factor Xa activity and thrombin generation in individuals treated with rivaroxaban and apixaban.

Designed as randomized, double blind, and placebo controlled, the ANNEXA trials (n = 145 healthy volunteers, ages 50–75 years) contained 2 arms: ANNEXA-R (rivaroxaban), and ANNEXA-A (apixaban).[37,59] To attain steady-state plasma levels, ANNEXA-R participants (n = 41) received 20 mg of rivaroxaban orally, once daily for 4 days, and ANNEXA-A subjects (n = 33) received 5 mg of apixaban orally, twice daily for 3.5 days. Participants received an 800-mg bolus of andexanet, and an 800-mg bolus followed by a continuous infusion of andexanet (8 mg/min for 120 minutes) with the endpoints of anti–factor Xa activity and thrombin generation.[37,59]

Rivaroxaban participants receiving andexanet therapy (n = 27) experienced a 92% decrease in anti–factor Xa activity, and a restoration of 96% of thrombin generation, as compared with an 18% decrease in anti–factor Xa activity ($P<.001$) and a 7% restoration of thrombin generation ($P<.001$) in participants who received placebo (n = 14).[59] In apixaban subjects, anti–factor Xa activity was decreased by 94%, and thrombin generation restored in 100% of individual having received andexanet (n = 24; a 21% decrease in anti–factor Xa activity; $P<.001$) and an 11% restoration of thrombin generation ($P<.001$) were observed among participants who received placebo (n = 9).[59] Given these findings, in May 2018, the FDA issued accelerated approval of andexanet alfa for use in patients experiencing life-threatening or uncontrolled bleeding occurring secondary to rivaroxaban and apixaban.[60]

An additional, ongoing trial that warrants mention is the ANNEXA-4: a multicenter, prospective, open-label, single-group study of andexanet given to patients treated with apixaban, rivaroxaban, edoxaban, and enoxaparin with acute major bleeding (defined as bleeding with severe hypotension, poor skin perfusion, mental confusion or low cardiac output; acute symptomatic retroperitoneal, intraarticular, pericardial, intracranial, or intramuscular bleeding with compartment syndrome; or overt bleeding with an acute decrease in hemoglobin of 2 g/dL or a hemoglobin of <8 g/dL if the baseline level is known).[61] All subjects were treated with an andexanet bolus followed by a 2-hour infusion. Primary outcomes were percent change in anti–factor Xa activity, and the rate of excellent or good hemostatic efficacy 12 hours after andexanet infusion.[61]

For intracranial hemorrhage, less than a 20% increase in volume at 12 hours, as determined by serial computed tomography scans or MRI, was considered excellent hemostasis.[59,61] Good hemostasis was classified as less than a 35% increase in volume at 12 hours.[59,61] Subarachnoid and subdural bleeds were classified in a similar manner, with an assessment of hematoma thickness.[58] Measurements of corrected hemoglobin and hematocrit at 12 hours after andexanet therapy were used to evaluate nonvisible bleeding.[61] A decrease in hemoglobin and hematocrit of less than 10% was considered excellent, whereas a decrease of less than 20% with the addition of no more than 2 units of blood products or coagulation therapies (eg, FFP or PCC) was considered good.[61] Cessation of visible bleeding within 1 hour of andexanet therapy was deemed excellent.[61] Good hemostatic efficacy was assigned if hemostasis was obtained within 4 hours of andexanet administration.[61] Pain relief, improvement in objective signs of bleeding, and the absence of an increase in swelling indicated excellent hemostatic efficacy if they occurred within 1 hour of infusion, and good if they occurred within 4 hours.[61]

In an interim analysis, 67 patients received andexanet (32 taking rivaroxaban [median daily dose 20 mg], 31 taking apixaban [median daily dose 5 mg], and 4 administered enoxaparin): 28 patients presented with intracranial bleeding, 33 with gastrointestinal bleeding, and 6 with bleeding at alternative sites.[61] Twenty patients were excluded from efficacy analysis (baseline anti–factor Xa below therapeutic anti-coagulation levels [n = 17], data were missing [n = 2], or enrollees did not meet the criteria for an acute major bleed [n = 3]).[61] In the efficacy population, among patients taking rivaroxaban (n = 26), anti–factor Xa activity was reduced by 89% (95% confidence interval, 58–94).[61] Anti–factor Xa activity decreased by 93% (95% confidence interval, 55–93) in patients treated with apixaban (n = 20), and the single patient in the efficacy group treated with enoxaparin had a reduction in anti–factor Xa activity from 0.61 IU/mL to 0.46 IU at 4 hours after bolus and infusion.[61]

Of the 47 patients in the efficacy population, 31 were determined to have excellent hemostasis and 6 good hemostasis (37 excellent or good hemostasis, 79% total efficacy population; 95% confidence interval, 64–89).[61] Of the 9 patients with poor or no hemostatic efficacy, 5 had been receiving rivaroxaban and 4 apixaban (4 with intracranial bleeding, 3 with gastrointestinal bleeding, and 2 with other sites of primary bleeding).[61] Subgroup analysis of the efficacy population revealed excellent or good efficacy for 80% of patients with intracranial bleeding and 84% of patients with gastrointestinal bleeding.[61] Of the 67 patients who received andexanet therapy, 12 experienced thrombotic events between 4 and 30 days of treatment (1 MI, 5 cerebrovascular accidents, 7 DVTs, and 1 PE).[61] Within the 30-day study period there were 10 deaths (6 cardiovascular, 4 noncardiovascular).[61] Because all patients had a history of thrombotic events and cardiovascular disease, it is unclear whether the frequency of these events exceeded those expected in this at risk population.[61] Additional data are required before making recommendations regarding the use of andexanet alfa.

Previous studies have evaluated the efficacy of rFVIIa, PCC, and FEIBA for the reversal of factor Xa inhibitors. In animal models, rFVIIa failed to reverse the anticoagulation effects of rivaroxaban.[62] In the previously discussed ex vivo study of 10 healthy male volunteers performed by Marlu and colleagues,[52] of the 3 therapies, only FEIBA was able to modify the quantitative and kinetic effects of rivaroxaban. In a randomized, double-blind, placebo-controlled study of 12 healthy male volunteers, a single bolus of 50 IU/kg PCC immediately and completely reversed the prolongation of the PT induced by 2.5 days of rivaroxaban therapy (20 mg orally, twice daily; $P<.001$).[63] Further studies are required to assess the efficacy of these therapies in patients experiencing bleeding events while taking factor Xa inhibitors. In the interim, the Hemostasis and Thrombosis Research Society deems the use of 4-factor PCC as a reasonable approach to the reversal of anticoagulation in this setting.[64]

Aripazine (PER977, Ciraparantag, Perosphere) is a synthetic molecule designed as a reversal agent for DTIs, factor Xa inhibitors, and unfractionated and low-molecular-weight heparin.[38,39] The mechanism of action of aripazine is poorly understood. In animal bleeding models (without anticoagulant therapy), this reversal agent has been demonstrated to reduce blood loss.[65,66] In animal studies involving novel oral anticoagulants (factor Xa inhibitors and dabigatran), aripazine administration reduced blood loss, and improved PT and aPTT.[67] A double-blinded, placebo-controlled trial involving 80 healthy male subjects treated with edoxaban (60 mg) revealed complete reversal of anticoagulation (measured in whole blood clotting time) within 10 to 30 minutes of the administration of 100 to 300 mg of aripazine.[68] Phase II clinical trials are now underway.[68] **Table 5** reviews reversal agents for factor Xa inhibitors.

Antifibrinolytic Agents

The efficacy of antifibrinolytic agents such as tranexamic acid and aminocaproic acid in direct oral anticoagulant-associated bleeding is unknown. because these agents are relatively inexpensive and possess favorable safety profiles, experts recommend that they be considered in the setting of life-threatening bleeding[69,70] (**Table 6**).

Table 5
Reversal agents for factor Xa inhibitors

Agent	Dose	Notes
Four-factor PCC (Kcentra)	25–50 U/kg	Repeat doses beyond 50 U/kg not advised. Maximum dose to be administered: 5000 U.
Factor VIII inhibitor-bypassing activity	50–100 U/kg	Repeat dosing may be considered after 6 h if significant bleeding persists.

Data from Refs.[12,64,85]

REVERSAL OF ANTIPLATELET THERAPY

Antiplatelet agents include aspirin, an irreversible inhibitor of cyclooxygenase-1 and cyclooxygenase-2; the thienopyridines, clopidogrel (Plavix; Bristol-Myers Squibb), prasurgrel (Effient; Eli Lilly, Bloomington, IN) and ticlopidine, which irreversibly inhibit the P2Y12 receptor for adenosine diphosphate on platelets; ticagrelor (Brilinta; AstraZeneca Pharmaceuticals, Cambridge, UK) and cangrelor (Kengreal, Chiesi Farmaceutici S.p.a., Parma, Italy), adenosine diphosphate receptor inhibitors; and dipyridamole, a reversible inhibitor of adenosine diphosphate uptake by platelets.[71–77] Antiplatelet therapy is used to prevent platelet aggregation and thrombosis in the setting of acute MI, non-ST segment elevation MI, and unstable angina.[71–77] Antiplatelet agents are also indicated for the prevention of ischemic cerebrovascular accidents, MIs, and death in patients who have experienced acute coronary syndrome, and for the prevention of stent thrombosis after percutaneous coronary intervention.[71–77]

Currently, there are no clinical practice guidelines that direct the treatment of life-threatening bleeding in the setting of antiplatelet therapy (save the discontinuation of all antiplatelet and anticoagulant agents). Although 1 in vitro model demonstrated drug-naïve platelet transfusion as effective in reversing platelet inhibition resulting from triple antiplatelet therapy (protease-activated receptor-1 antagonist [inhibits thrombin-induced platelet aggregation] plus dual antiplatelet therapy),[78] the PATCH (Platelet Transfusion versus Standard Care after Acute Stroke due to Spontaneous Cerebral Haemorrhage Associated with Antiplatelet Therapy) trial demonstrated

Table 6
Antifibrinolytic agents

Agent	Dose	Notes
Tranexamic acid	1 g IV	Requires dosing adjustment for renal impairment.
Aminocarproic acid	4–5 g IV infusion during the first hour of treatment followed by 1 g/h for 8 h or until control of bleeding.	Rapid IV administration should be avoided: may induce hypotension, bradycardia, or arrhythmia.

Abbreviation: IV, intravenous.

Data from US Food and Drug Administration. Highlights of prescribing information: CYKLOKAPRON® (tranexamic acid injection). Available at: https://www.accessdata.fda.gov/drugsatfda_docs/label/2011/019281s030lbl.pdf. Accessed December 25, 2017; and US Food and Drug Administration (FDA). Highlights of prescribing information: AMICAR® Injection. Available at: https://www.accessdata.fda.gov/drugsatfda_docs/label/2004/15197scm036,scf037,scp038,scm039_amicar_lbl.pdf. Accessed December 25, 2017.

Table 7 Reversal agents for platelet inhibitors		
Agent	**Dose**	**Notes**
Platelets	2–3 apheresis units or 2–3 units of pooled platelets	Human studies have failed to demonstrate morbidity and mortality reduction following administration.
Desmopressin (DDAVP)	0.4 μg/kg IV	Consider in addition to platelet transfusion.

From Frontera J, Lewin J III, Rabinstein A, et al. Guideline for reversal of antithrombotics in intracranial hemorrhage. Neurocrit Care 2016;24(1):6–46; with permission.

platelet transfusion for spontaneous intracranial hemorrhage as ineffective in the reduction of bleeding, and associated with increased mortality within 3 months after adminstration.[79] At this point in time, further research is required before making recommendations regarding platelet transfusion for the reversal of antiplatelet therapy.[80]

Desmopressin (Stimate; CSL Behring), or DDAVP, is a synthetic analogue of antidiuretic hormone, indicated for the treatment of bleeding episodes in persons with type I von Willebrand disease, or hemophilia A patients with greater than 5% factor VIII activity.[81] A recent metaanalysis of 10 randomized controlled trials (n = 596 participants undergoing cardiac surgery) revealed that individuals treated with desmopressin were transfused fewer red cells, had less blood loss, and had a lower risk of reoperation owing to bleeding; however, the quality of this evidence was low to moderate, suggesting uncertainty regarding the effect of desmopressin in patients with recent antiplatelet drug administration.[82] Despite this finding, current guidelines from the Neurocritical Care Society and Society of Critical Care Medicine support the use of a one-time 0.3 μg/kg intravenous dose of desmopressin in patients receiving antiplatelet therapy who experience intracranial hemorrhage[83] **(Table 7)**.

SUMMARY

Anticoagulants are now the most common outpatient pharmaceutical therapy associated with adverse drug events.[84] Among individuals age 65 and older, warfarin, dabigatran, rivaroxaban, and enoxaparin account for nearly 60% of drug-related emergency department visits, and in 2016 alone (most recent FDA Adverse Event Reporting System data), hemorrhage secondary to anticoagulant therapy resulted in the death of more than 3000 individuals.[84] As an ever increasing number of Americans are prescribed warfarin, direct oral anticoagulants, and antiplatelet therapies, it is essential that the emergency physician is equipped to address bleeding complications.

REFERENCES

1. Office of Disease Prevention and Health Promotion. National action plan for adverse drug event prevention. Available at: https://health.gov/hcq/pdfs/ADE-Action-Plan-Anticoagulants.pdf. Accessed January 3, 2018.

2. Barnes G, Lucas E, Alexander G, et al. National trends in ambulatory oral anticoagulant use. Am J Med 2015;128:1300–5.

3. Kumar V, Abbas A, Fausto N, et al. Hemodynamic disorders, thromboembolic disease and shock. In: Kumar V, Abbas A, Aster J, editors. Robbins and Cotran: pathologic basis of disease. 9th edition. Philadelphia: Elsevier Saunders; 2015. p. 116–22.
4. Paniccia R, Priora R, Liotta A, et al. Platelet function tests: a comparative review. Vasc Health Risk Manag 2015;11:133–48.
5. Porteus M, Mantanona T. Chapter 14. blood. In: Janson LW, Tischler ME, editors. The big picture: medical biochemistry. New York: McGraw-Hill; 2012. p. 213–9.
6. US Food and Drug Administration (FDA). Highlights of prescribing information: Coumadin® tablets (warfarin sodium tablets, USP), Coumadin® for injection (warfarin sodium for injection, USP). Available at: http://www.accessdata.fda.gov/drugsatfda_docs/label/2010/009218s108lbl.pdf. Accessed December 29, 2017.
7. Gonsalves W, Pruthi R, Patnaik M. The new oral anticoagulants in clinical practice. Mayo Clin Proc 2013;88(7):777.
8. Herzog E, Kaspereit F, Krege W, et al. Four-factor prothrombin complex concentrate (4F-PCC) is superior to three-factor prothrombin complex concentrate (3F-PCC) for reversal of coumarin anticoagulation. Blood 2014; 124:1472.
9. Harter K, Levine M, Henderson S. Anticoagulation drug therapy: a review. West J Emerg Med 2015;16(1):11–7.
10. US Food and Drug Administration (FDA). Highlights of prescribing information: Profilnine. Available at: http://www.fda.gov/ucm/groups/fdagov-public/@fdagov-bio-gen/documents/document/ucm261964.pdf. Accessed December 29, 2017.
11. Holland L, Warkentin T, Refaai M, et al. Suboptimal effect of a three-factor prothrombin complex concentrate (Profilnine-SD) in correcting supratherapeutic International Normalized Ratio due to warfarin overdose. Transfusion 2009;49(6): 1171–7.
12. US Food and Drug Administration (FDA). Highlights of prescribing information: KCENTRA. Available at: https://www.fda.gov/ucm/groups/fdagov-public/@fdagov-bio-gen/documents/document/ucm350239.pdf. Accessed December 29, 2017.
13. US Food and Drug Administration (FDA). Highlights of prescribing information: FEIBA. Available at: https://www.fda.gov/downloads/BiologicsBloodVaccines/BloodBloodProducts/ApprovedProducts/LicensedProductsBLAs/FractionatedPlasmaProducts/UCM221749.pdf. Accessed January 3, 2018.
14. Zareh M, Davis A, Henderson S. Reversal of warfarin-induced hemorrhage in the emergency department. West J Emerg Med 2011;12(4):386–92.
15. Wójcik C, Schymik M, Cure E. Activated prothrombin complex concentrate factor VIII inhibitor bypassing activity (FEIBA) for the reversal of warfarin-induced coagulopathy. Int J Emerg Med 2009;2(4):217–25.
16. Sarode R, Milling T, Refaai M, et al. Efficacy and safety of a 4-factor prothrombin complex concentrate in patients on vitamin K antagonists presenting with major bleeding: a randomized, plasma-controlled, Phase IIIb study. Circulation 2013; 128(11):1234–43.
17. Milling T, Refaai M, Goldstein J, et al. Thromboembolic events after vitamin K antagonist reversal with 4-factor prothrombin complex concentrate: exploratory analyses of two randomized, plasma-controlled studies. Ann Emerg Med 2016; 67(1):96–105.
18. Aledort L. Comparative thrombotic event incidence after infusion of recombinant factor VIIa versus factor VIII inhibitor bypass activity. J Thromb Haemost 2004; 2(10):1700–8.

19. Awad N, Cocchio C. Activated prothrombin complex concentrates for reversal of anticoagulant-associated coagulopathy. P T 2013;38(11):696–701.
20. Hickey M, Gatien M, Taljaard M, et al. Outcomes of urgent warfarin reversal with frozen plasma versus prothrombin complex concentrate in the emergency department. Circulation 2013;128(4):360–4.
21. Nee R, Doppenschmidt D, Donovan D, et al. Intravenous versus subcutaneous vitamin K in reversing excessive oral anticoagulation. Am J Cardiol 1999;83: 286–8.
22. Bechtel B, Nunez T, Lyon J, et al. Treatments for reversing warfarin anticoagulation in patients with acute intracranial hemorrhage: a structured literature review. Int J Emerg Med 2011;4:40.
23. Steiner T, Rosand J, Diringer M. Intracerebral hemorrhage associated with oral anticoagulant therapy: current practices and unresolved questions. Stroke 2006;37:256–62.
24. US Food and Drug Administration (FDA). Novo Nordisk. Novo Seven: coagulation factor VIIa (recombinant) for intravenous use only. Available at: https://www.fda.gov/downloads/.../ucm056915.pdf. Accessed January 4, 2018.
25. MacLaren R, Weber L, Brake H, et al. A multicenter assessment of recombinant factor VIIa off-label usage: clinical experiences and associated outcomes. Transfusion 2005;45(9):1434.
26. Hoots W. Challenges in the therapeutic use of a "so-called" universal hemostatic agent: recombinant factor VIIa. Hematology Am Soc Hematol Educ Program 2006;426–31.
27. US Food and Drug Administration (FDA). Heparin sodium injection, USP. Available at: https://www.accessdata.fda.gov/drugsatfda_docs/label/2006/017037s158lbl.pdf. Accessed January 3, 2018.
28. US Food and Drug Administration (FDA). Highlights of prescribing information: Lovenox (enoxaparin sodium injection) for subcutaneous and intravenous use. Available at: https://www.accessdata.fda.gov/drugsatfda_docs/label/2009/020164s085lbl.pdf. Accessed January 3, 2018.
29. US Food and Drug Administration (FDA). Highlights of prescribing information: Fragmin (dalteparin sodium injection) for subcutaneous use only). Available at: https://www.accessdata.fda.gov/drugsatfda_docs/label/2010/020287s050lbl.pdf. Accessed January 3, 2018.
30. US Food and Drug Administration (FDA). Arixtra (fondaparinux sodium) injection. Available at: https://www.accessdata.fda.gov/drugsatfda_docs/label/2005/021345s010lbl.pdf. Accessed January 3, 2018.
31. Eikelboom J, Hirsh J. Monitoring unfractionated heparin with the aPTT: time for a fresh look. Thromb Haemost 2006;96(5):547–52.
32. Babin J, Traylor K, Witt D. Laboratory monitoring of low-molecular-weight heparin and fondaparinux. Semin Thromb Hemost 2017;43(4):261–9.
33. Alnie N, Reston R, Jenkins P, et al. Protamine sulfate down-regulates thrombin generation by inhibiting factor V activation. Blood 2009;114(8):1658–65.
34. Weber JE, Jaggi FM, Pollack CV. Anticoagulants, antiplatelet agents, and fibrinolytics. In: Tintinalli JE, Kelen GD, Stapczynski JS, editors. Emergency medicine: a comprehensive study guide. 6th edition. McGraw-Hill; 2004. p. 1354–60.
35. van Veen JJ, Maclean RM, Hampton KK, et al. Protamine reversal of low molecular weight heparin: clinically effective? Blood Coagul Fibrinolysis 2011;22: 565–70.
36. Glangarande P. Fondaparinux (Arixtra): a new anticoagulant. Int J Clin Pract 2002;56(8):615–7.

37. Kaatz S, Bhansali H, Gibbs J, et al. Reversing factor Xa inhibitors – clinical utility of andexanet alfa. J Blood Med 2017;8:141–9.
38. Hu T, Vaidya V, Asirvatham S. Reversing anticoagulant effects of novel oral anti-coagulants: role of ciraparantag, andexanet alfa, and idarucizumab. Vasc Health Risk Manag 2016;12:35–44.
39. Abo-Salem E, Becker R. Reversal of novel oral anticoagulants. Curr Opin Pharmacol 2016;27:86–91.
40. Ansell J, Laulicht B, Hoffman M, et al. Ciraparantag safely and completely reverses the anticoagulant effects of low molecular weight heparin. Thromb Res 2016;146:113–8.
41. US Food and Drug Administration (FDA). Highlights of prescribing information: Pradaxa® (dabigatran etexilate mesylate) capsules, for oral use. Available at: https://www.accessdata.fda.gov/drugsatfda_docs/label/2015/022512s028lbl.pdf. Accessed December 23, 2017.
42. Rhea J, Molinaro R. Direct thrombin inhibitors: clinical uses, mechanism of action, and laboratory measurement. MLO Med Lab Obs 2011;43(8):20, 22, 24.
43. Weitz J, Hirsh H, Samama M. New antithrombotic drugs: American College of Chest Physicians Evidence-Based Clinical Practice Guidelines ((8th edition. Chest 2008;133(6 Suppl):234S–56S.
44. Wann L, Curtis A, Ellenbogen K, et al. ACC/AHA/HRS focused update on the management of patients with atrial fibrillation (update on Dabigatran): a report of the American College of Cardiology Foundation/American Heart Association Task Force on Practice Guidelines. Circulation 2011;123(10):1144–50.
45. US National Library of Medicine. Randomized evaluation of long term anticoagulant therapy (RE-LY) with Dabigatran Etexilate. Available at: https://clinicaltrials.gov/ct2/show/results/NCT00262600. Accessed December 23, 2017.
46. US Food and Drug Administration (FDA). Highlights of prescribing information: Praxbind® (idarucizumab) injection, for intravenous use. Available at: https://www.accessdata.fda.gov/drugsatfda_docs/label/2015/761025lbl.pdf. Accessed December 24, 2017.
47. Pollack C, Reilly P, van Ryn J, et al. Idarucizumab for dabigatran reversal-full cohort analysis. N Engl J Med 2017;377:431–41.
48. Pallack C, Reilly P, Weitz J. correspondence: authors' reply: dabigatran reversal with idarucizumab. N Engl J Med 2017;377:1690–2.
49. Getta B, Muller N, Motum P, et al. Intermittent haemodialysis and continuous veno-venous dialysis are effective in mitigating major bleeding due to dabigatran. Br J Haematol 2015;169(4):603–4.
50. Sarich T, Seltzer J, Berkowitz S, et al. Novel oral anticoagulants and reversal agents: considerations for clinical development. Am Heart J 2015;169(6):751–7.
51. Cuker A, Siegal D. Monitoring and reversal of direct oral anticoagulants. Hematology Am Soc Hematol Educ Program 2015;2015:117–24.
52. Marlu R, Hodaj E, Albaladejo P, et al. Effect of non-specific reversal agents on anticoagulant activity of dabigatran and rivaroxaban: a randomized crossover ex vivo study in healthy volunteers. Thromb Haemost 2013;109(1):169.
53. US Food and Drug Administration (FDA). Highlights of prescribing information: XARELTO (rivaroxaban) tablets, for oral use. Available at: https://www.accessdata.fda.gov/drugsatfda_docs/label/2011/202439s001lbl.pdf. Accessed December 24, 2017.
54. US Food and Drug Administration (FDA). Highlights of prescribing information: ELIQUIS (apixaban) tablets for oral use. Available at: https://www.accessdata.

fda.gov/drugsatfda_docs/label/2012/202155s000lbl.pdf. Accessed December 24, 2017.

55. US Food and Drug Administration (FDA). Highlights of prescribing information: SAVAYSA (edoxaban) tablets for oral use. Available at: https://www.accessdata.fda.gov/drugsatfda_docs/label/2015/206316lbl.pdf. Accessed December 24, 2017.

56. US Food and Drug Administration (FDA). Highlights of prescribing information: BEV-YXXA (betrixaban) capsules, for oral use. Available at: https://www.accessdata.fda.gov/drugsatfda_docs/label/2017/208383s000lbl.pdf. Accessed January 4, 2018.

57. Cuker A, Siegal D, Crowther M, et al. Laboratory measurement of the anticoagulant activity of target-specific oral anticoagulant agents: a systematic review. J Am Coll Cardiol 2014;64(11):1128–39.

58. Noll A. Expert analysis: coagulation assays and the new oral anticoagulants. American College of Cardiology, Latest in Cardiology; 2015. Available at: http://www.acc.org/latest-in-cardiology/articles/2015/06/22/12/06/coagulation-assays-and-the-new-oral-anticoagulants. Accessed December 24, 2017.

59. Siegal D, Curnutte J, Connolly S, et al. Andexanet alfa for the reversal of factor Xa inhibitor activity. N Engl J Med 2015;373(25):2413–24.

60. US Food and Drug Administration (FDA). Accelerated Approval: Portola Pharmaceuticals. Available at: https://www.fda.gov/downloads/BiologicsBloodVaccines/CellularGeneTherapyProducts/ApprovedProducts/UCM606693.pdf. Accessed June 22, 2018.

61. Connolly S, Milling T, Elkelboom J, et al. Andexanet alfa for acute major bleeding associated with factor Xa inhibitors. N Engl J Med 2016;375:1131–41.

62. Gruber A, Marezec U, Buetehorn U, et al. Potential of activated complex concentrate and activated factor VII to reverse anticoagulant effects of rivaroxaban in primates. Haematologica 2009;92(Suppl2):181.

63. Eerenberg E, Kamphuisen P, Sijpkens M, et al. Reversal of rivaroxaban and dabigatran by prothrombin complex concentrate: a randomized, placebo-controlled, crossover study in healthy subjects. Circulation 2011;124:1573–9.

64. Kaatz S, Kouides P, Garcia D. Guidance on the emergent reversal of oral thrombin and factor Xa inhibitors. Am J Hematol 2012;87(Suppl 1):S141–5.

65. Hollenbach S, Lu G, DeGuzman F, et al. Andexanet-alfa and PER977 (aripazine) correct blood loss in rabbit liver laceration model. Circulation 2014;130:A14657.

66. Lu G, Kotha J, Cardenas J, et al. In vitro characterization of andexanet alfa (PRT064445), a specific fXa inhibitor antidote versus aripazine (PER977), a non-specific reversal agent. Circulation 2014;130:A18218.

67. Laulicht B, Bakhru S, Lee C, et al. Small molecule antidote for anticoagulants. Circulation 2012;126:A11395.

68. Ansell J, Bakhru S, Laulicht B, et al. Single-dose cirapantag safely and completely reverses anticoagulant effects of edoxaban. Thromb Haemost 2017;117(2):238–45.

69. Weitz J, Pollack C. Practical management of bleeding in patients receiving non-vitamin K antagonist oral anticoagulants. Thromb Haemost 2015;114(6):1113–26.

70. Pollack C. Coagulation assessment with the new generation of oral anticoagulants. Emerg Med J 2016;33(6):423–30.

71. US Food and Drug Administration (FDA). Aspirin: comprehensive prescribing information. Available at: https://www.fda.gov/ohrms/dockets/ac/03/briefing/4012B1_03_Appd%201-Professional%20Labeling.pdf. Accessed January 4, 2018.

72. US Food and Drug Administration (FDA). Plavix clopidogrel bisulfate tablets. Available at: https://www.accessdata.fda.gov/drugsatfda_docs/label/2009/020839s044lbl.pdf. Accessed January 4, 2018.
73. US Food and Drug Administration (FDA). TICLID® (ticlopidine hydrochloride). Available at: https://www.accessdata.fda.gov/drugsatfda_docs/nda/2001/19-979S018_Ticlid_prntlbl.pdf. Accessed January 4, 2018.
74. US Food and Drug Administration (FDA). Highlights of prescribing information: EFFIENT (prasugrel) tablets. Available at: https://www.accessdata.fda.gov/drugsatfda_docs/label/2010/022307s002lbl.pdf. Accessed January 4, 2018.
75. US Food and Drug Administration (FDA). Highlights of prescribing information: BRILINTA®. Available at: https://www.accessdata.fda.gov/drugsatfda_docs/label/2016/022433s020lbl.pdf. Accessed January 4, 2018.
76. US Food and Drug Administration (FDA). Highlights of prescribing information: KENGREAL™(cangrelor) for injection, for intravenous use. Available at: https://www.accessdata.fda.gov/drugsatfda_docs/label/2015/204958lbl.pdf. Accessed January 4, 2018.
77. US Food and Drug Administration (FDA). Drugs@FDA: FDA approved drug products: persantine. Available at: https://www.accessdata.fda.gov/scripts/cder/daf/index.cfm?event=overview.process&ApplNo=012836. Accessed January 4, 2018.
78. Bhal V, Herr M, Dixon M, et al. Platelet function recovery following exposure to triple anti-platelet inhibitors using an in vitro transfusion model. Thromb Res 2015;136(6):1216–23.
79. Baharoglu M, Cordonnier C, Al-Shahi Salman R, et al. Platelet transfusion versus standard care after acute stroke due to spontaneous cerebral haemorrhage associated with antiplatelet therapy (PATCH): a randomised, open-label, phase 3 trial. Lancet 2016;387(10038):2605–13.
80. Kaufman R, Djulbegovic B, Gernsheimer T, et al. Platelet transfusion: a clinical practice guideline from the AABB. Ann Intern Med 2015;162(3):205–13.
81. U.S Food and Drug Administration (FDA). Stimate® (desmopressin acetate). Available at: https://www.accessdata.fda.gov/drugsatfda_docs/label/2011/020355s013lbl.pdf. Accessed January 4, 2018.
82. Desborough M, Oakland K, Landoni G, et al. Desmopressin for treatment of platelet dysfunction and reversal of antiplatelet agents: a systematic review and meta-analysis of randomized controlled trials. J Thromb Haemost 2017;15(2):263–72.
83. Frontera J, Lewin J III, Rabinstein A, et al. Guideline for reversal of antithrombotics in intracranial hemorrhage. Neurocrit Care 2016;24(1):6–46.
84. Shehab N, Lovegrove M, Geller A, et al. US Emergency department visits for outpatient adverse drug events, 2013-2014. JAMA 2016;316(20):2115–25.
85. US Food and Drug Administration (FDA). Highlights of prescribing information: KCENTRA (prothrombin complex concentrate (human)). Available at: https://www.fda.gov/ucm/groups/fdagov-public/@fdagov-bio-gen/documents/document/ucm350239.pdf. Accessed December 25, 2017.

Rapid Fire: Acute Blast Crisis/Hyperviscosity Syndrome

Geremiha Emerson, MD*, Colin G. Kaide, MD

KEYWORDS

- Blast • Leukostasis • Leukapheresis • Petechiae • Hyperviscosity
- Chronic myeloid leukemia • Acute myeloid leukemia • Hydroxyurea

KEY POINTS

- Blast crisis is usually seen in patients with acute and chronic myeloid leukemia.
- Clinical manifestations of blast crisis involve bone marrow infiltration (eg, anemia, thrombocytopenia, bleeding, bone pain, and immunosuppression) and hyperleukocytosis.
- Leukostasis is defined by symptomatic hyperleukocytosis with neurologic and/or pulmonary manifestations.
- DIC, tumor lysis syndrome, and leukostasis can happen in patients with hyperleukocytosis.
- Most cases of leukocytosis will have white blood cell counts greater than 100,000 with greater than 20% blast cells.

CASE: SHORTNESS OF BREATH

Pertinent History: The patient is a 45 year-old man presenting with several days of shortness of breath, cough, and low-grade fevers (up to 100.5°F). It is associated with a generalized headache that was gradual in onset, as well as generalized fatigue and malaise. He denies any associated chest pain, confusion, lethargy, nausea, vomiting, or diarrhea. He reports a gradual overall decline in his function over the last several weeks; he is currently able to complete only a few blocks of his usual daily 5-mile runs. He presents to the emergency department for evaluation of a possible cardiac cause of his symptoms. He denies tobacco or illicit drug use. He has no known past medical history and is currently on no medications (**Fig. 1**).

Pertinent Physical Examination: Blood pressure is 145/95. Pulse is 95; RR is 30, and SpO2 is 87%. Temperature is 100.5°F.

General: The patient appears in mild distress.
Head, eyes, ears, nose, and throat: Gingival petechiae.

Disclosure Statement: The authors have no disclosures.
Department of Emergency Medicine, Wexner Medical Center at The Ohio State University, 760 Prior Hall, 376 West 10th Avenue, Columbus, OH 43210, USA
* Corresponding author.
E-mail address: Geremiha.Emerson@osumc.edu

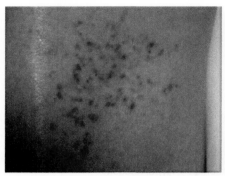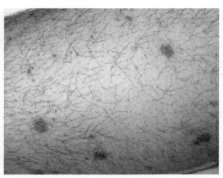

Fig. 1. Petechiae. (*Courtesy of* C. Kaide, MD, Wexner Medical Center at The Ohio State University, Columbus, Ohio, USA.)

Neck: Supple. No meningismus.
Cardiovascular: Regular rate and rhythm. No murmurs, rubs or gallops.
Pulmonary/Chest: Crackles in all fields.
Abdominal: Non-tender, non-distended.
Neuro: Alert and oriented x3. Delayed reciprocity in speech. No focal weakness.
Skin: Scattered petechiae.
Extremities: No deformities.

Diagnostic testing: laboratory testing results were

WBC: 450K (99% Blasts)
HbB: 8.5
Plt: 23K
Na: 135
K: 5.8
HCO_3: 22
BUN: 35
Cr: 3.2
Ca: 6.4
PO_4: 5.5
LDH: 600
Uric Acid: 6.2

Chest radiograph showed bilateral interstitial infiltrates.
Computed tomography of the chest showed bilateral parenchymal infiltrates and ground glass opacities. There were no pulmonary emboli.
Diagnosis is acute blast crisis with leukostasis.
The plan is volume expansion with intravenous fluids, STAT hematology consultation for leukaphoresis, admission, and chemotherapy.

LEARNING POINTS: BLAST CRISIS AND HYPERVISCOSITY (LEUKOSTASIS)
Introduction/Background

1. Blast crisis is (variably) defined by the presence of greater than 20% of peripheral or bone marrow blast cells. Blast cells refer to early hematopoietic cells from the lymphoid (lymphocytes) or myeloid (erythrocytes, thrombocytes, monocytes, neutrophils, basophils, eosinophils) cell lines. Healthy bone marrow should contain no more than 5% blast cells. Normal peripheral blood should contain no blasts (**Fig. 2**)

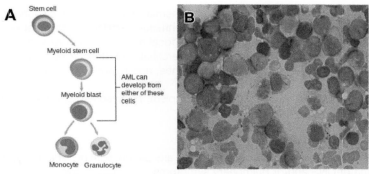

Fig. 2. (*A*) Blast cells. (*B*) Blasts on peripheral smear. (*Courtesy of* [*A*] Cancer Research UK/Wikimedia Commons; and *From* [*B*] Wikipedia Commons (https://commons.wikimedia.org/wiki/File: Myeloblast_with_Auer_rod_smear_2010-01-27.JPG), "Myeloblast with Auer rod smear 2010-01-27", https://creativecommons.org/licenses/by-sa/3.0/legalcode. Accessed February 1, 2018.)

2. Two main underlying factors seem to lead to hyperleukocytosis. First, the rapid proliferation of blasts within the bone marrow leads to a large tumor burden. Second, normal hematopoietic cell adhesion becomes disrupted and leads to a reduced affinity to the bone marrow.[1]
3. Clinical manifestations of blast crisis can be divided into 2 major categories. The first category includes complications that result from bone marrow infiltration. These include anemia, thrombocytopenia, bleeding, bone pain, and immunosuppression. The second category includes complications related to extremely elevated (>50–100,000) peripheral white blood cell counts (hyperleukocytosis).
4. Hyperleukocytosis manifests in 3 main problems: leukostasis, disseminated intervascular coagulation (DIC) and tumor lysis syndrome. This review will focus on leukostasis.
   a. Leukostasis, also known as symptomatic hyperleukocytosis, is an acute hematologic emergency. It is defined hyperleukocytosis with neurologic and/or pulmonary manifestations.[2] It is most commonly seen in patients with acute myeloid leukemia (AML) and chronic myeloid leukemia (CML). Although less common, it can also be seen in acute or chronic lymphocytic leukemia (ALL or CLL).[2] It generally occurs with higher total leukocyte counts, often exceeding 100,000.[2]
   b. Systemic microvascular obstruction and endothelial activation can lead to DIC, which can be seen in varying degrees in up to 40% of patients with acute leukostasis.[2]
   c. Spontaneous tumor lysis syndrome is seen in about 10% of patients suffering from leukostasis.[1]

Pathophysiology

1. The pathophysiology of leukostasis is incompletely understood, and is likely the result of multiple factors. These include
   a. Increasing volumes of relatively rigid blast cells leads to microvessel occlusion and decreased blood flow. The end result is tissue ischemia.
   b. Endothelial activation by inflammatory cytokines released by blast cells results in increased adhesion of blast cells to the endothelium.[3]
   c. Local endothelial hypoxia induced by high metabolic demands of rapidly dividing blast cells results in endothelial damage and malfunction.[3]
2. Microvascular obstruction and endothelial damage lead to tissue hypoxia and organ dysfunction. The most common sites for symptomatic microvascular obstruction include the CNS and the lungs.[4]

a. CNS manifestations include focal ischemia, edema, and occasionally hemorrhage. Signs and symptoms include confusion, headache, ataxia, blurred vision, altered/depressed mental status, and focal numbness and weakness.
b. Pulmonary manifestations include interstitial and alveolar edema and hemorrhage. This leads to dyspnea, tachypnea, and hypoxemia. Rales can often be appreciated on auscultation.
c. Additional manifestations include priapism, limb ischemia, renal insufficiency, and renal vein thrombosis.

Making the Diagnosis

1. Acute leukostasis should be suspected in any patient with hyperleukocytosis complaining of CNS and/or pulmonary symptoms.
2. Laboratory testing should include comprehensive blood count with differential, comprehensive metabolic panel, coagulation studies, and a uric acid level.
    a. Most cases of leukocytosis with have WBC greater than 100,000 with greater than 20% blast cells.[2]
    b. Anemia and thrombocytopenia are common.
    c. Evidence of concomitant DIC includes coagulopathy, decreased fibrinogen, and elevated D-dimer.
    d. Evidence of tumor lysis includes hyperkalemia, hyperphosphatemia, hypocalcemia, and elevated uric acid.
        i. Pseudohyperkalemia as a result of in vitro cell lysis after blood draw is commonly seen in hyperleukocytosis. Whole blood samples obtained via blood gas analysis can provide more accurate potassium measurements in this setting.[5]
3. Imaging studies can provide support for the diagnosis of leukostasis, although findings are nonspecific. CNS imaging may demonstrate edema, infarction, or hemorrhage. Pulmonary imaging may demonstrate interstitial and/or alveolar infiltrates[2] (**Box 1**, **Fig. 3**).

Treating the Patient

1. Early recognition and consideration of associated complication are the most important aspects of the emergency department management of patients with leukostasis. Emergent hematology consultation is essential as soon as leukostasis is suspected. The ultimate goal is for rapid reduction of peripheral WBC count, which is accomplished by emergent leukophoresis and/or chemotherapy.[1,6–8]
    a. Patients with asymptomatic hyperleukocytosis may be treated with hydroxyurea.[1]

Box 1
Leukostasis manifestations

Organ Involved	Manifestations
Lung	Shortness of breath, hypoxia, diffuse alveolar hemorrhage
CNS	Confusion, altered mentation, focal neurologic deficits, headache, delirium
Vascular system	Ischemia of limbs, venal vein thrombosis, priapism
Heart	Myocardial infarction
Eye/Ear	Vision changes, retinal hemorrhage/tinnitus

The presence of any of these manifestations in the right context may indicate leukostasis.[1]

Courtesy of C. Kaide, MD, Wexner Medical Center at The Ohio State University, Columbus, Ohio, USA.

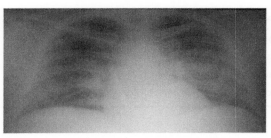

Fig. 3. Chest radiograph showing pulmonary vascular congestion. (*Courtesy of* Colin Kaide, MD, Columbus, Ohio, USA; with permission.)

2. Volume expansion with intravenous fluids can help provide a degree of hemodilution and improved viscosity. Patients with leukostasis often have a clinical picture similar to volume overload (dyspnea, interstitial/alveolar infiltrates on chest radiograph). Careful consideration should be taken before withholding intravenous fluids, as most patients are likely not volume overloaded and may benefit from the dilutional effect of fluids.[2]
3. Consider early administration of broad-spectrum antibiotics if infection is suspected. These patients are likely immunosuppressed, as blasts are nonfunctional white cells. Fever is commonly seen in patients with leukostasis (up to 80%), although this may be the result of blast cell cytokine release rather than infection.[1]
4. Thrombocytopenia may be the result of bone marrow suppression or DIC. Early platelet transfusion should be done to maintain platelet count greater than 20,000 to 30,000 in order to reduce the risk of serious bleeding, including intracranial hemorrhage.
5. Red blood cell transfusion should be avoided unless absolutely necessary, as it is likely to increase viscosity and worsen leukostasis.[2]
6. If emergent leukophoresis or chemotherapy is not immediately available, therapeutic phlebotomy (500–1000 mL) followed by aggressive volume expansion can temporize while arrangements are made for transfer to definitive management.[2]

CASE SUMMARY

The patient was admitted to the intensive care unit (ICU), where emergent leukophoresis was initiated. Pathology returned with acute myeloid leukemia. The patent was initiated on induction chemotherapy with cytarabine and daunorubicin. He showed excellent clinical response and was ultimately discharged home. Final diagnosis was acute myeloid leukemia with blast crisis and leukostasis.

CASE DISCUSSION

These observations are made based on these writers' experience with blast crisis and leukostasis. Acute blast crisis with leukostasis is a rare complication of hematologic malignancies. Symptoms are variable and typically vague, requiring a high index of suspicion to make the diagnosis. Suspect leukostasis in any patient presenting with hyperleukocytosis. Early identification and definitive management are essential. Involve consultants early. If definitive management (eg, leukophoresis or chemotherapy) and/or expert care are not available, early transfer is essential for survival.

Pattern Recognition
• Hyperleukocytosis
• Vague symptoms
• CNS and/or pulmonary manifestations
• Subacute symptoms with rapid decompensation

REFERENCES

1. Röllig C, Ehninger G. How I treat hyperleukocytosis in acute myeloid leukemia. Blood 2015;125:3246–52.
2. Porcu P, Cripe LD, Ng EW, et al. Hyperleukocytic leukemias and leukostasis: a review of pathophysiology, clinical presentation and management. Leuk Lymphoma 2000;39:1.
3. Stucki A, Rivier AS, Gikic M, et al. Endothelial cell activation by myeloblasts: molecular mechanisms of leukostasis and leukemic cell dissemination. Blood 2001; 97:2121.
4. Azoulay E, Fieux F, Moreau D, et al. Acute monocytic leukemia presenting as acute respiratory failure. Am J Respir Crit Care Med 2003;167:1329.
5. Bellevue R, Dosik H, Spergel G, et al. Pseudohyperkalemia and extreme leukocytosis. J Lab Clin Med 1975;85(4):660–4.
6. Bug G, Anargyrou K, Tonn T, et al. Impact of leukapheresis on early death rate in adult acute myeloid leukemia presenting with hyperleukocytosis. Transfusion 2007; 47:1843.
7. Porcu P, Farag S, Marcucci G, et al. Leukocytoreduction for acute leukemia. Ther Apher 2002;6:15.
8. Marbello L, Ricci F, Nosari AM, et al. Outcome of hyperleukocytic adult acute myeloid leukaemia: a single-center retrospective study and review of literature. Leuk Res 2008;32(8):1221–7.

Emergency Medicine Evaluation and Management of Anemia

Brit Long, MD[a],*, Alex Koyfman, MD[b]

KEYWORDS

- Anemia • Red blood cells • Evaluation • Management • Microcytic • Normocytic
- Macrocytic • Transfusion • Transfusion reaction

KEY POINTS

- Anemia is commonly found on laboratory evaluation and is due to decreased red blood cells or hemoglobin concentration. Definition varies based on age.
- Anemia can be broken into several types based on symptoms, time of onset, and red blood cell indices (using MCV with microcytic, normocytic, and macrocytic).
- Transfusion considerations include assessment of patient hemodynamics. Unstable patients with anemia require transfusion.
- A transfusion threshold of 7 g/dL is recommended for patients with sepsis, trauma, critical illness, and gastrointestinal bleeding.
- Iron is an alternative treatment for patients with microcytic anemia owing to iron deficiency, and hyperbaric oxygen therapy is another option if available.

INTRODUCTION

Anemia is common in the emergency department (ED), frequently diagnosed on laboratory evaluation. Emergency physicians play an integral role in the diagnosis and management of anemia. Patients may demonstrate a wide variety of symptoms, with many remaining relatively asymptomatic. Few patients require acute intervention in the ED; however, significant variation is present in the management of anemia.[1–6] Understanding the different types of anemia and treatment modalities may improve ED evaluation and management of this common condition.

Disclosure Statement: This review does not reflect the views of opinions of the U.S. government, Department of Defense, U.S. Army, U.S. Air Force, or SAUSHEC EM Residency Program.
[a] Department of Emergency Medicine, San Antonio Military Medical Center, 3841 Roger Brooke Drive, Fort Sam Houston, TX 78234, USA; [b] Department of Emergency Medicine, The University of Texas Southwestern Medical Center, 5323 Harry Hines Boulevard, Dallas, TX 75390, USA
* Corresponding author.
E-mail address: brit.long@yahoo.com

Emerg Med Clin N Am 36 (2018) 609–630
https://doi.org/10.1016/j.emc.2018.04.009
0733-8627/18/Published by Elsevier Inc.

emed.theclinics.com

DEFINITION OF ANEMIA

Anemia is a condition in which the body has decreased erythrocytes, otherwise known as red blood cells (RBCs), which is measured as a decreased hemoglobin concentration.[2–5] Hemoglobin levels of less than 13 g/dL in adult males and 12 g/dL in adult females define anemia according to the World Health Organization.[2,4] The definition of anemia can also include the lowest 2.5% of hemoglobin levels in a healthy population.[5,6] Normal hemoglobin and hematocrit levels depend on several factors, especially age and gender (**Table 1**).

EPIDEMIOLOGY

Anemia affects approximately 25% of the world's population and is more commonly found in children, females, the elderly, and chronically ill patients.[2,7–9] Women and African Americans at baseline have lower hemoglobin levels.[6,10] In the United States, the prevalence decreases to less than 5%, although more than 30% of patients older than 85 years demonstrate anemia.[7–17] Anemia is not a normal component of aging, with risk factors including male gender, nutritional deficiencies, advancing age, and chronic disease.[16,17] Anemia occurs in one-half of pregnant patients in the world, although this is 20% in the United States.[2,18] The risk in the United States increases with lower socioeconomic status, nutritional issues, and chronic illness.[7–11] Anemia can affect quality of life and may contribute to all-cause mortality in elderly patients, as well as increase the risk of fall and functional impairment.[9,11,19–23] Chronic anemia may lead to congestive heart failure or cardiovascular disease if severe.[2,15,16] From a practical perspective, there are only three possible causes of anemia: decreased RBC production, blood loss, and increased RBC destruction.

ERYTHROPOIESIS

An RBC functions to transport oxygen from the lungs to the rest of the body and carbon dioxide to the lungs for removal. The bone marrow is the originator of several cell lines, including RBCs after several cell divisions. RBCs are discoid, pliable cells containing four hemoglobin molecules but no nucleus. Erythropoietin, a glycoprotein from renal peritubular cells, controls RBC production.[1–5] RBC production requires erythropoietin stimulus, precursor cells within the bone marrow, and nutrients for synthesis.[5,24–28] Normal formation of RBCs requires 3 to 7 days. A normoblast is the originator that extrudes a nucleus to form a reticulocyte. This reticulocyte matures into an RBC with loss of the ribosomal network. The normal lifespan of an RBC is 100 to 120 days before the cell is removed by macrophages.[5,24–28]

Abnormalities in the production of RBCs can result in anemia, and these abnormalities can be the result of vitamin deficiency (vitamin B_{12} or folate) or a genetic hemoglobinopathy or membranopathy. Hemoglobinopathies are the result of

Table 1 Normal hemoglobin and hematocrit levels by age and gender		
Age	Hemoglobin (g/dL)	Hematocrit (mL/dL)
≤3 mo	10.4–12.2	30–36
3–7 y	11.7–13.5	34–40
Adult female	12.0–16.0	35–48
Adult male	14.0–18.0	40–52

abnormal hemoglobin (sickle cell anemia and thalassemia), whereas membranopathies are associated with abnormalities in the RBC membrane, such as hereditary spherocytosis.[2,5,13]

HEMOGLOBIN

Hemoglobin carries oxygen and consists of two pairs of polypeptide chains, each with a heme complex for oxygen binding along the iron molecule. The major and minor forms of hemoglobin are hemoglobin A and A2. Hemoglobin F (the most common form in utero) is also present, which makes up less than 2% of hemoglobin in normal adults. This form can be higher in patients with hemoglobin variants.[5,13] The environment and genetics affect the structure of hemoglobin and the overall oxygen-carrying capacity.[2,5,24] Patients with sickle cell disease possess hemoglobin S predominantly. Hemoglobin C and E and thalassemia are other abnormal forms of hemoglobin. These variant forms generally result in a shorter RBC life span, altered affinity for oxygen, and an increased tendency toward hemolysis. An altered ability of hemoglobin to carry oxygen occurs with carbon monoxide toxicity, methemoglobinemia, sulfhemoglobinemia, and cyanohemoglobinemia.[2,5,13]

The body normally maintains a constant mass of RBCs, as reticulocytes replace the removed RBCs. In the presence of anemia, the body responds in several ways depending on degree of anemia, rapidity of onset, and patient condition.[24–28] Acute onset of anemia (commonly from intravascular blood loss) often results in vasoconstriction peripherally with blood flow preferentially directed to key organ systems, such as the heart, lungs, brain, and kidneys. RBCs increase their ability to release oxygen to tissues in these states.[2,13,29,30] If chronic anemia is present, plasma volume increases to maintain overall blood volume. Erythropoietin also increases owing to chronic tissue hypoxia, resulting in increased production within the bone marrow and release of immature RBCs, known as reticulocytes.[2,5,24–28]

In chronic anemia, hemoglobin levels approaching 5 to 6 g/dL may be safe in certain populations owing to several adaptations. Several studies suggest physiologic compensatory mechanisms can optimize peripheral oxygen delivery.[2,5,30,31] Patients with chronic anemia experience a change in 2,3-DPG levels, allowing greater release of oxygen from hemoglobin to peripheral tissues, along with increased cardiac output.[2,5,30,31]

TYPES

Anemia is classified in several ways, although in the ED acute versus chronic is the easiest means of differentiation.[2,5,24]

Acute Anemia

Acute anemia causes include hemorrhage from trauma, gastrointestinal (GI) blood loss, aneurysm rupture, and genitourinary bleeding.[2,5] It is also important to remember that, in patients who have had a recent catheterization procedure with access via the groin, retroperitoneal hemorrhage can be an occult source of life-threatening bleeding. Sickle cell disease with aplastic crisis and acute splenic or hepatic sequestration can result in acute anemia. Microangiopathic hemolytic anemias and disseminated intravascular coagulation are other etiologies of acute anemia.[32] Dilutional anemia occurs with rapid crystalloid infusion.

Chronic Anemia

Chronic anemia is defined by the specific etiology with RBC destruction or decreased RBC production. The determination of several RBC indices, such as mean corpuscular volume (MCV), provides further assistance in characterization.[2,5,11,24] Chronic anemia is most commonly due to iron deficiency and anemia of chronic disease.[2,5,11]

EVALUATION

Anemia possesses a wide spectrum of signs and symptoms. Patients with evidence of hemodynamic instability believed to be due to hemorrhage require active stabilization and resuscitation, followed by a more thorough history and examination.[2,5,33–35]

FEATURES

Manifestations of anemia depend on the rate of decrease in hemoglobin and the patient's compensation. The oxygen-carrying capacity of RBCs exceeds oxygen tissue needs by a factor of four at rest.[30,34–38] If the patient has documented anemia, the physician should evaluate for blood loss of the GI, genitourinary, or pulmonary systems, which are the three most common systems involved in hemorrhage.[2,5] A thorough history regarding menstruation for women and hematemesis, hemoptysis, hematuria, hematochezia, and melena should be obtained. Past medical history, procedures and surgeries, medications, diet (folate, B_{12}, iron intake), and family history (sickle cell, glucose-6-phosphate deficiency, spherocytosis) can provide important clues to anemia.[2,5,11] Medications associated with anemia include aspirin, angiotensin-converting enzyme inhibitors, angiotensin receptor blockers, bisphosphonates, carbamazepine, cephalosporins, nonsteroidal anti-inflammatory drugs, phenytoin, sulfa drugs, and chemotherapy agents.[39–42]

The presentation of anemia includes weakness, fatigue, irritability, headache, decreased exercise tolerance, palpitations, dyspnea, and potentially angina over a more chronic period owing to compensation.[2,5,11] These patients usually do not display evidence of acute bleeding. Patients commonly do not develop symptoms unless the hemoglobin level decreases to less than 7 g/dL, although no specific level is definitive for symptoms.[30,35,36] Patients with forms of chronic anemia such as sickle cell disease may demonstrate a baseline level of 5 to 6 g/dL.[2,5,11,13]

Signs of acute blood loss associated with emergent anemia can include hemodynamic abnormalities such as hypotension, tachycardia, and tachypnea, and the patient may experience decreased urine output, increased thirst, and altered mental status.[29,33,34] These clinical manifestations depend on several factors such as patient comorbidities, age, baseline medications, and severity of illness or injury. For example, younger adults may demonstrate an ability to compensate with an increased heart rate. However, older patients with baseline medical problems more commonly are unable to compensate.[5,9] This may be especially true if they are chronically on beta-blockers.

Examination is often normal in patients with chronic anemia, although several findings are suggestive of certain causes.[32,39] Pallor, scleral icterus, and jaundice are associated with hemolytic anemia. Physicians should assess for evidence of cardiac murmur, crackles, hepatomegaly or splenomegaly, thyromegaly, and lymphadenopathy.[2,5] Evaluation for tenderness, joint deformities, rashes, and melena or blood on rectal examination is important. Evidence of bleeding with chronic anemia suggests a coagulation disorder.[35,36,43] As discussed, patients can adapt to low hemoglobin levels such as 5 to 6 g/dL if anemia is slow in onset.

LABORATORY ASSESSMET

Laboratory evaluation of the patient with anemia can provide valuable information. These tests include a complete blood count, peripheral smear, reticulocyte count, type and screen (type and crossmatch if transfusing in the ED), coagulation assessment (prothrombin time/International Normalized Ratio, partial thromboplastin time), electrolyte panel, creatinine level, urinalysis, lactate dehydrogenase, haptoglobin, and uric acid.[2,5,6,11,32,44,45]

Complete Blood Count

The hemoglobin, hematocrit, and RBC value provide the initial diagnosis of anemia. In acute hemorrhage, it may take hours before a baseline is established, and laboratory assessment during active hemorrhage may reveal initially normal values. Spectrophotometry directly measures hemoglobin, and the hematocrit and RBC values are calculated from this measure.[2,6,45] Point-of-care testing measures hematocrit through conductivity analysis, although test accuracy depends on normal physiology. Values of less than 30% may result in inaccurate testing.[2,5,11,40]

The complete blood count often displays RBC indices to assist with an anemia diagnosis. These values are show in in **Table 2**, which discusses hemoglobin, hematocrit, RBC distribution width, MCV, mean cell hemoglobin, and mean cell hemoglobin concentration.[2,5,6]

Peripheral Smear

A peripheral smear is usually obtained if abnormal RBCs are detected on the complete blood count. This test allows for an assessment of RBC shape and abnormal cells present in the blood. Peripheral smear findings are helpful in suggesting specific disease states (**Table 3**). Schistocytes are associated with thrombotic microangiopathies.[2,5,6,32,45]

Other Assessments

Several laboratory tests are useful in further differentiating the underlying etiology of anemia. Reticulocytes, or immature RBCs, are found in states with accelerated RBC production. Values greater than 1.5% in men and 2.5% in women are defined as elevated. Normal hemoglobin level and elevated reticulocyte count suggest polycythemia. The reticulocyte count is typically elevated in anemia if the bone marrow is responding appropriately. The reticulocyte index is calculated by (reticulocyte count [%] × [patient hematocrit/normal hematocrit])/2. An index of greater than 2 is

Table 2 Hemoglobin, hematocrit, RDW		
Parameter	**Definition**	**Normal Value (Male, Female)**
Hgb	Determined by spectrophotometry, refers to concentration of hemoglobin	14–18, 12–16
Hematocrit	Calculated from Hgb, often 3× greater	40–52, 35–47
RDW	Measure of RBC size variation	11.5%–14.5%
MCV	Space taken up by RBCs in plasma, calculated by (hematocrit × 10)/RBC count	80–100
MCH	Calculated by (hemoglobin × 10)/RBC count	26–34 pg
MCHC	Calculated by (hemoglobin × 100)/hematocrit	31%–36%

Abbreviations: Hgb, hemoglobin; MCH, mean cell hemoglobin; MCHC, mean cell hemoglobin concentration; MCV, mean corpuscular volume; RBC, red blood cells; RDW, red blood cell distribution width.

Table 3
Peripheral smear findings

Finding in Smear	Disease Associated with Finding
Burr cells	Microangiopathic hemolytic anemia, renal disease
Clumping	Presence of cold antibodies
Rouleaux formation	Multiple myeloma, inflammatory state, Waldenstrom macroglobulinemia
Schistocyte	Hemolysis, microangiopathic hemolytic anemia
Sickle cells	Sickle cell disease
Spherocytes	Hereditary spherocytosis, autoimmune hemolytic anemia
Target cells (codocytes)	Hemoglobinopathies, iron deficiency
Teardrop cells (dacrocytes)	Leukoerythroblastic syndrome

appropriate. An index of less than 2 suggests abnormal bone marrow response.[2,5,27,28,45,46] Hemolysis can elevate bilirubin (typically indirect), blood urea nitrogen, and creatinine. A blood urea nitrogen/creatinine ratio of more than 30 is suggestive of upper GI bleeding. Elevated creatinine is associated with renal disease.[2,5,46] RBC destruction results in release of lactate dehydrogenase that, if elevated, suggests hemolytic anemia. Haptoglobin (normal values 36–195 mg/dL) functions as an acute phase reactant with a half-life of 5 days.[2,5,11,32,47] This molecule binds to free hemoglobin, which is quickly cleared from serum. Decreased haptoglobin suggest hemolysis. A Coombs tests consist of direct and indirect globulin tests.[32,39,46,47] A positive direct globulin test suggests erythrocyte membrane antibodies, indicating autoimmune hemolytic anemia.[32,39,46,47] An indirect Coombs test evaluates for free minor antibodies against RBCs in the serum and is used in pretransfusion testing.

Microcytic anemia can be due to iron deficiency, which is assessed with four assays: serum iron, ferritin, transferrin, and total iron-binding capacity. Macrocytic anemia can be due to a variety of factors, and assessment of B_{12}, folate, and thyroid-stimulating hormone is warranted.[2,5,11,13]

APPROACH

The patient with hemodynamic instability owing to hemorrhage requires resuscitation with transfused blood products. In a hemodynamically stable patient with newly diagnosed anemia, the physician should evaluate RBC indices, peripheral smear, and reticulocyte index. RBC indices of greater than 2 suggest appropriate bone marrow response, whereas values of less than 2 are inappropriate. The MCV is one of the first indices helpful for diagnosis, with values of less than 80 as microcytic and values of greater than 100 macrocytic (**Table 4**). These values assist in determining the underlying etiology.[2,5,11,13]

Microcytic Anemia

An MCV of less than 80 is defined as microcytic anemia, which is most commonly due to iron deficiency (iron deficiency anemia [IDA]), followed by thalassemia and anemia of chronic disease. A ferritin of less than 15 mg/L is 99% specific for IDA, and if ferritin is normal or high, thalassemia or anemia of chronic disease is likely.[4,27,28,44] Microcytic anemia with a ferritin of less than 15 mg/L is diagnostic

Table 4 MCV for diagnosing anemia		
Class	**MCV**	**Causes**
Microcytic	<80	Iron deficiency Anemia of chronic disease: vasculitis, chronic heart or renal failure, chronic infection Sideroblastic anemia Lead toxicity Thalassemia: alpha and beta
Normocytic	80–100	Renal disease Autoimmune: viral, drug, idiopathic, vasculitis Hemolytic anemia: sickle cell disease, glucose-6-phosphate deficiency, spherocytosis, elliptocytosis Microangiopathic Infection: bacterial, malaria, parvovirus, babesiosis Endocrine gland failure (not including thyroid)
Macrocytic	> 100	Megaloblastic: vitamin B_{12} or folate deficiency Inhibitors of DNA synthesis Myelodysplasia Chronic liver disease Reticulocytosis Hypothyroidism Failure of bone marrow

Abbreviation: MCV, mean corpuscular volume.

of IDA. However, ferritin may still be normal in IDA. Transferrin saturation of less than 20% in the setting of normal or slightly low ferritin is also diagnostic of IDA.[4,27,28,44] Low prior hemoglobin values with low MCV suggests a congenital disorder such as alpha or beta thalassemia. Asymptomatic mild anemia associated with beta thalassemia minor in the Mediterranean population is often confused with IDA. Of note, anemia of chronic disease may be microcytic or normocytic, and sideroblastic anemia, an acquired or hereditary bone marrow disorder, may present in a similar manner (sideroblastic anemia will have high RBC distribution width values).[24,25]

Normocytic

Normocytic anemia is defined by an MCV of 80 to 100, and several studies including reticulocyte count can be used to determine the etiology. Normal reticulocyte values are more commonly associated with microcytic or macrocytic anemia. A high reticulocyte value should be followed with a Coombs tests for further differentiation. RBC distribution width is also helpful, because normal values in the setting of normocytic anemia suggest chronic disease or renal failure (a creatinine of 1.5 mg/dL can result in anemia).[3,11,28,32]

Hemolytic anemia from RBC destruction is one of the most common causes of normocytic anemia. Several diseases resulting in hemolytic anemia can be deadly. Laboratory assessments such as increased indirect bilirubin, schistocytes on peripheral smear, elevated lactate dehydrogenase, elevated reticulocyte count, and decreased haptoglobin are suggestive. The differential includes disseminated intravascular coagulation, thrombotic thrombocytopenic purpura, hemolytic uremic syndrome, and preeclampsia/eclampsia. A positive Coombs test is suggestive of an autoimmune hemolytic anemia, whereas a negative Coombs tests is associated with RBC membrane defects or microangiopathic hemolysis.[3,32,39] Types of hemolytic anemias are presented in **Table 5**.

Table 5
Hemolytic anemias

Anemia	Signs and Symptoms	Underlying Etiology	Laboratory Tests	Management
DIC	Purpura, bleeding, thrombosis, end organ failure	Inflammation, severe disease	Elevated PT/PTT/INR/D-dimer, low fibrinogen, thrombocytopenia	Treat underlying disorder Transfuse platelets, FFP, cryoprecipitate
HUS	Bloody diarrhea, abdominal pain, acute renal injury	Infection with enterohemorrhagic *Escherichia coli*	Thrombocytopenia, schistocytes, normal coagulation panel	Supportive therapy, may require dialysis
TTP	Fever, CNS abnormalities/seizure, renal injury	ADATMS13 deficiency	Thrombocytopenia, schistocytes, normal coagulation panel	Plasma exchange, FFP
Warm AIHA	Depends on anemia severity	Autoantibodies against RBCs	Normal coagulation panel and platelets, +DAT, spherocytes	Steroid therapy

Abbreviations: AIHA, autoimmune hemolytic anemia; CNS, central nervous system; DIC, disseminated intravascular coagulation; FFP, fresh frozen plasma; HUS, hemolytic uremic syndrome; INR, International Normalized Ratio; PT, prothrombin time; PTT, partial thromboplastin time; RBCs, red blood cells; TTP, thrombotic thrombocytopenic purpura.

Macrocytic Anemia

This class consists of an MCV of greater than 100 and is divided into megaloblastic anemia, which is a result of poor erythropoiesis, and nonmegaloblastic anemia. The most common causes of macrocytic anemia include nutritional deficiency (folate and vitamin B_{12}), resulting in megaloblastic anemia, or specific drugs and toxins, most commonly causing nonmegaloblastic anemia.[2,5,44,48,49] Evaluation of these patients requires close consideration of current toxins or drugs such as chemotherapy agents, alcohol, hydroxyurea, and zidovudine.[44,48] Pernicious anemia is rarely the cause and is associated with gastric intrinsic factor deficiency. Vitamin B_{12} and folate levels can assist, although they possess low sensitivity and specificity for definitive diagnosis. Folate levels can rapidly change with dietary modification and be falsely elevated in states of low vitamin B_{12}. If a low folate level is discovered, RBC folate and homocysteine (HC) levels should be evaluated. RBC folate levels will be low and HC levels elevated in folate deficiency. Vitamin B_{12} deficiency is usually caused by poor nutrition resulting from either low intake or poor absorption. Serum B_{12} may be falsely low in patients with multiple myeloma, leukopenia, pregnancy, and oral contraceptive use. Normal vitamin B_{12} levels cannot exclude the diagnosis. Diagnosis requires methylmalonic acid and HC levels, which will be elevated in vitamin B_{12} deficiency, although methylmalonic acid is more sensitive than HC. In folate deficiency, methylmalonic acid is normal and HC elevated.[2,5,11,13,44,48,49]

Other etiologies include primary bone marrow disease, associated with macrocytosis, liver disease, and hypothyroidism. A peripheral smear to assess for target cells (liver disease) and a thyroid assessment are recommended (**Fig. 1**).[2,5,11,13,44,48,49]

GENERAL MANAGEMENT

The management of the patient with anemia focuses primarily on patient clinical status, along with the primary etiology. The first, and most vital, question centers on need for blood transfusion. This decision should not be taken lightly, because transfusion is associated with risks including infection and transfusion reactions.[33,34]

The Unstable Patient

Patients who are hemodynamically unstable owing to anemia or hemorrhage require resuscitation, with control of the source of bleeding. The physician should seek sites of external trauma or hemorrhage. If discovered on primary or secondary physical examination, direct pressure and reversal are needed.[2,29,34] The absence of trauma requires consideration of internal hemorrhage, primarily GI, genitourinary, pulmonary, and retroperitoneal in the right circumstances. Physical examination may assist, but further studies such as imaging with ultrasound examination, computed tomography scans, or endoscopy may definitively find the source of hemorrhage. Consultation with surgery, gastroenterology, or interventional radiology may be required.[2,29,34]

Although evaluating the source of bleeding and stopping ongoing hemorrhage are essential, patients with hemodynamic instability require blood product transfusion. No specific hemoglobin/hematocrit level is recommended for patients with active hemorrhage. Crystalloids should be used sparingly to improve cardiac preload, but these fluids will dilute oxygen-carrying capacity.[2,5,29,33,34] Uncrossmatched RBCs, O-positive in male and postmenopausal female patients, and O-negative in female patients of reproductive age, should be emergently provided. A type and crossmatch should be sent immediately, and once fully crossmatched blood

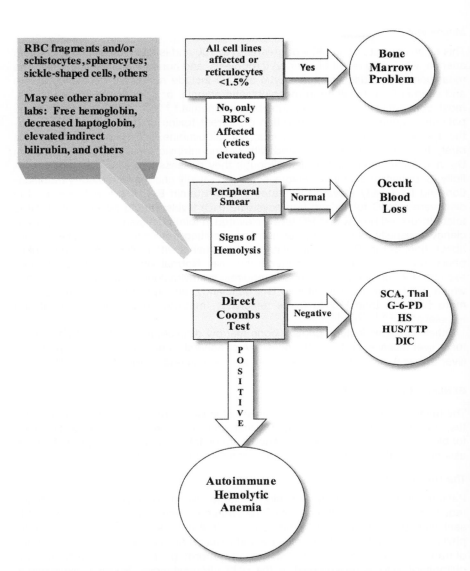

Fig. 1. Simplified approach to anemia without obvious source of blood loss. DIC, disseminated intravascular coagulation; HS, hereditary spherocytosis; HUS, hemolytic uremic syndrome; SCA, sickle cell anemia; TTP, thrombotic thrombocytopenic purpura. (*Courtesy of* C. Kaide, MD, Wexner Medical Center at The Ohio State University, Ohio.)

is available, it should be given.[2,29,50,51] Patients requiring multiple units of blood may need massive transfusion protocol with fresh frozen plasma and platelets as well.[50,51]

The Stable Patient

Patients who are hemodynamically stable with anemia may require no further assessment or treatment.[2,5,11,13] This state is determined by several other important factors, including patient comorbidities, the underlying etiology of the anemia, the ability to follow-up, and the presence of symptoms.

Transfusion

Tissue oxygenation depends on hemoglobin concentration and saturation, oxygen supply, cardiac output, and pulmonary function.[33,34,52–54] Transfusion targets improvement in these factors. More than 15 million units of blood products are transfused annually in the United States, and close to 40% of patients in intensive care receive a transfusion.[34,54–57] A single unit donated from whole blood provides close to 2 units of packed RBCs (pRBCs), which are stored between 1°C and 6°C with adenine, citrate, phosphate, and dextrose.[2,33,56,57] One unit of RBCs elevates hemoglobin by 1 g/dL and hematocrit by 3%.[58–61] RBCs can improve hemoglobin concentration, oxygen delivery to tissues, and cardiac output. However, it may also increase blood viscosity and diminish peripheral oxygen delivery owing to RBC storage defects. RBCs are normally stored for up to 42 days, and storage may increase RBC deformities, increase cytokines, and decrease 2,3-diphosphoglycerate (2,3-DPG).[33,56–59] However, the literature suggests transfusion of fresher pRBCs is not superior to pRBCs stored up to 42 days with regard to mortality.[33,34]

The clinical situation, patient's hemodynamic status, intravascular volume, and comorbidities should be considered when determining need for transfusion. Patients with critical illness demonstrate decreased erythropoietin production, increased cytokine production, and iron deficiency, all of which contribute to anemia.

A specific, universally accepted transfusion threshold is elusive, with multiple guidelines in use. Originally, transfusion for hemodynamically stable patients was recommended for hemoglobin/hematocrit of less than 10/30. This value was first suggested in 1942.[62–64] This specific threshold was used for several populations with anemia. More recent literature, however, recommends against this level. Lower transfusion thresholds (often referred to as "restrictive strategy") including a hemoglobin of 7 to 8 g/dL have been demonstrated to be safe in several patient populations.[33,34] One of the first studies demonstrating this was the 1999 Transfusion Requirements in Critical Care (TRICC) trial, which was performed in patients in intensive care with a hemoglobin of less than 9 g/dL.[34,65] No difference in all-cause mortality was found between patients randomized to 7 or 10 g/dL, although mortality during hospitalization was improved in the restrictive group.[65] A 2012 Cochrane review suggests a lower transfusion threshold reduces in-hospital mortality, but may not affect duration of stay or patient recovery.[66,67] More recent meta-analyses report less total mortality, acute coronary syndrome (ACS), pulmonary edema, and bacterial infection risk in patients with a restrictive transfusion strategy, as opposed to liberal transfusion.[68,69]

Sepsis

For sepsis, the original transfusion threshold of 10/30 (hemoglobin/hematocrit) was questioned by The Transfusion Requirements in Septic Shock (TRISS) trial, finding patients in the 7 g/dL threshold group had fewer units transfused but no change in mortality, ventilator support, or vasopressor support.[34,70] More recent trials have used this threshold of 7 g/dL with no change in mortality or other patient-centered outcomes.[71,72] This level is safe in patients with sepsis, severe sepsis, and septic shock.

Gastrointestinal Bleeding

Patients with GI bleeding also benefit from a 7 g/dL threshold.[33,34] Villanueva and colleagues[73] randomized patients with GI bleeding to 7 g/dL versus 9 g/dL, finding lower mortality and bleeding rates in the lower threshold group. Patients with active exsanguination were excluded, however. Other studies suggest similar outcomes with reduced mortality, duration of stay, and less transfusion in restrictive groups.[34,74,75]

Trauma

Patients actively hemorrhaging in the setting of trauma require emergent transfusion, preferably with 1:1:1 (massive transfusion protocol) if more than 4 U pRBCs will be given.[34,50,51,76] Trauma patients who do not require massive transfusion may benefit from restrictive strategy with a threshold for transfusion 7 g/dL, with literature suggesting decreased rates of mortality and multiple organ dysfunction with 7 g/dL when compared with 10 g/dL.[34,77] Infection risk increases with greater number of units transfused.[78–80]

Acute Coronary Syndrome

Patients with ACS present greater controversy for transfusion thresholds.[2,33,34] Myocardial oxygen demand is higher in ACS. This demand must be balanced against circulatory overload and increased thrombogenicity, which can worsen with transfusion.[34,81] Several studies suggest decreased cardiac events and death with a higher transfusion threshold,[82,83] whereas others suggest improved mortality with decreased transfusion.[84,85] A meta-analysis suggests a number needed to harm of 8 for transfusion in ACS. Studies in these populations suffer from significant biases and confounders.[85] In a hemodynamically stable patient, transfusion threshold of 7 to 8 g/dL is likely safe.[2,33,34]

Neurologic Disease

Transfusion in patients with traumatic brain injury or other conditions such as subarachnoid hemorrhage is also controversial; studies suggest a threshold of 8 to 9 g/dL.[86–90] A subgroup analysis of the TRICC trial found no mortality difference between 7 g/dL and 10 g/dL,[89] and a meta-analysis suggested no difference between 6 g/dL and 10 g/dL.[90]

In summary, for patients who are not critically ill with no cardiovascular disease, a level of 7 g/dL is recommended. Critically ill patients, including those with sepsis, GI bleeding, and trauma, can also be transfused at 7 g/dL.[2,33,34] However, evidence of active exsanguination or hemodynamic instability may require transfusion. Elderly patients and those with heart disease may benefit from a threshold of 8 g/dL, especially if patients have symptoms consistent with ischemic heart disease (chest pain, shortness of breath).[33,34]

Table 6 American Association of Blood Banks transfusion guidelines	
Recommendation	**Evidence Grade**
Transfusion is not indicated in hemodynamically stable hospitalized patients (including critically ill patients) until the Hgb level is 7 g/dL, rather than 10 g/dL	Strong recommendation, moderate quality evidence
For patients with cardiovascular disease or those receiving orthopedic or cardiac surgery, a transfusion threshold of 8 g/dL is recommended	Strong recommendation, moderate quality evidence
All patients can receive pRBCs within their licensed dating period rather than limiting patients to only fresh pRBCs (such as those <10 d)	Strong recommendation, moderate quality evidence

Abbreviations: Hgb, hemoglobin; pRBCs, packed red blood cells.
From Carson JL, Guyatt G, Heddle NM, et al. Clinical practice guidelines from the AABB red blood cell transfusion thresholds and storage. JAMA 2016;316(19):2025–35.

TRANSFUSION REACTIONS

Transfusion is a major procedure with several risks. Physicians should consider the clinical situation and potential harms and benefits of transfusion. Several different reactions are possible, one of which is alloimmunization among Rh(−) reproductive-aged women.[33,34] The rate of alloimmunization reaches 8% per product transfused, which results in RBC antibodies that may cross the placenta in future pregnancies, potentially resulting in hemolytic disease of the newborn.[33,34] Other risks are shown in **Table 6**. Although patients are often most concerned with risk of infection, this risk is actually low, with hepatitis C at 1 in 1,149,000, hepatitis B at 1 in 1,200,000, and human immunodeficiency virus at 1 in 1,467,000 (**Table 7**).[33,34,91–98]

ALTERNATIVES TO TRANSFUSION

Several alternatives to transfusion are available. The American Society of Anesthesiologists recommends no transfusion if the following are present: the patient is young and healthy, no ongoing bleeding is present, and hemoglobin is greater than 6 g/dL.[99] Fatigue, pallor, and reduced exercise tolerance are not indications for blood product transfusion, although chest pain, shortness of breath, and evidence of hemodynamic instability are stronger indications for transfusion.[11,99–102] If IDA is present, iron therapy can be efficacious, well-tolerated, and cost effective. Several iron preparations are available, although the most common is ferrous sulfate 300 to 325 mg, taken 3 to 4 times per day with food.[99–102] Vitamin C supplementation can also increase oral iron absorption.[99–112] Iron can be given to patients with IDA, especially in reproductive aged females who have primary care follow-up. However, other patients including pediatric, male, and older patients require further evaluation for the cause of IDA.[2,5,11,13] Depending on the specific type of anemia, erythropoietic growth factor, vitamin B_{12}, or folate supplementation can be used for management.[103]

Patients with poor oral absorption (gastric bypass, celiac disease), an inability to tolerate oral iron, a high rate of bleeding, and severe anemia with ongoing bleeding may benefit from intravenous (IV) iron.[101,104,105] Systemic infection, allergy, and prior hypotensive reaction to IV iron are contraindications.[101,103–105] The main risks of IV iron supplementation include hypotension (1%–2%), which is more frequent in patients older than 65 years and those with a low baseline systolic blood pressure, asthma, respiratory or cardiac disease, patients on antihypertensive medications, and chronic kidney disease.[101–105] More common adverse effects include myalgias, polyarthralgia, headache, chest discomfort, nausea, vomiting, and diarrhea. These symptoms typically resolve within 1 day after the infusion. Serious allergic reactions including anaphylaxis occur in fewer than 1 in 1,000,000 patients.[101,102]

IV iron is available in several forms: iron sucrose (300 mg in 250 mL of NS given over 2 hours) and ferumoxytol (510 mg in 17 mL with 50 mL NS, given over 15–60 minutes).[101,102] Oral iron supplementation daily is recommended after IV iron. Hemoglobin levels typically increase by 2 to 3 g/dL approximately 2 to 4 weeks after IV infusion.[101,102] IV iron is an option for preoperative patients, even in patients with cardiac disease, compared with transfusion.[99,101,102,113]

Another alternative to blood product transfusion includes normobaric or hyperbaric oxygen therapy, especially in patients with anemia who may not receive blood products owing to religious, immunologic, or personal reasons.[106–109] This therapy corrects oxygen debt in anemia while avoiding the potential risks of transfusion, although it requires a dive chamber and a hyperbaric medicine department. This equipment is not available in most centers. Pulsed, intermittent normobaric oxygen

Table 7
Transfusion reactions

Reaction	Pathophysiology	Symptoms	Occurrence (Units Transfused)
Febrile nonhemolytic reaction	Patient antibodies react with product antigens, as well as product cytokines.	Fever, usually low grade. Resolves with acetaminophen.	1:60–100
Bacterial infection	Products create medium for bacterial growth. Highest risk with platelets.	High fever, chills, hypotension, rigor, nausea/vomiting.	1:250,000
Allergic	Owing to product proteins/antigens, most common in patients with IgA deficiency.	Urticaria, pruritis, hypotension, nausea/vomiting. May meet criteria for anaphylaxis.	1:250–333
Acute hemolytic reaction	Product ABO incompatibility results in immune reaction and hemolysis.	Symptoms of anaphylaxis with hypotension, tachycardia, confusion, arrhythmia, shock, cardiac arrest, dyspnea.	1:250,000–600,000
Transfusion-associated acute lung injury (TRALI)	Transfused cytokines interact with patient blood cells, including WBCs.	Acute respiratory distress with fever, pulmonary edema, hypotension. Symptoms within 2–8 h.	1:5000–12,000
Transfusion associated circulatory overload (TACO)	Symptoms consistent with fluid overload: edema, dyspnea, orthopnea, hypertension.	Volume overload seen in patients with impaired cardiac function.	1:100
Delayed hemolytic reaction	Patient produces antibodies to RBC antigens, decreasing RBC survival.	Fever, jaundice, darkened urine; often subclinical reaction with minimal symptoms.	Unknown
Transfusion-associated graft-versus-host disease (GVHD)	Transfused cells attack patient cells, most often in immunosuppressed patients.	Many presentations, ranging from anaphylaxis to tachycardia, fever, and hypotension; may be fatal.	1:100–1000 in patients with malignancy
Iron overload	One unit of transfused RBC contains 2 mg of iron. Threshold of clinically significant iron overload likely at 10–20 U of RBC transfused.	Endocrine and liver dysfunction, cardiotoxicity, congestive heart failure, dysrhythmia.	Unknown

Abbreviations: IgA, immunoglobulin A; RBCs, red blood cells; WBCs, white blood cells.

therapy or hyperbaric therapy can increase RBC and hemoglobin mass. Hyperbaric therapy is administered by providing pressures at 2 to 3 atm absolute for 3 to 4 hours 3 to 4 times per day. The patient should be euvolemic, and a hemantinic is recommended to supplement RBC increase, along with nutritional support. This therapy is safe and comparable in cost with 1 U of pRBCs, with few and infrequent side effects.[106–109] Evidence suggests it is useful as a rescue intervention, but further study is required before routine use is recommended (**Box 1**).[106–109]

SPECIAL POPULATIONS
Pediatric Patients

Anemia affects close to 20% of US children.[1,2,110–112] Normal hemoglobin levels depend on age, with a normal physiologic nadir at 6 to 8 weeks of age, which increases to 9 g/dL.[2,5,11,13,110] Routine screening is not recommended for pediatric patients unless risk factors are present.[110–112,114] Anemia may be found incidentally, with a rate of occult anemia approaching 14% in 1 pediatric ED study.[115] However, anemia is not normal in pediatric patients, and further evaluation is required including RBC indices. Anemia in pediatric patients is commonly due to decreased production or increased destruction. Disorders such as sickle cell anemia and thalassemia require consideration.[1,2,110–112,114]

Geriatric Patients

Anemia is not physiologically normal in geriatric patients.[17,27,116,117] However, anemia is common in this population, ranging from 8% to 44%, and is even higher in patients older than 85 years.[17,27,116,117] The most common causes of anemia are anemia of chronic disease (30%–45%) and IDA (15%–30%).[117–123] Patients more commonly

---

Box 1
Why HBO therapy works

HBO therapy involves the exposure of the entire body to 100% oxygen at a pressure of greater than 1 atm absolute (ATA). This is accomplished in a hyperbaric chamber with the patient breathing 100% oxygen.

Under normobaric conditions, humans live under the downward pressure exerted by the weight of the atmosphere. This pressure is usually measured in millimeters of mercury (mm Hg). At sea level, 1 atm (ATA) is 760 mm Hg (14.7 lbs/in^2, 760 Torr). Under hyperbaric treatment conditions, the body is exposed to pressures that are typically in the range of 2.0 to 3.0 ATA—1 atmosphere from the earth's atmosphere plus an additional 1 to 2 atm exerted by pressurizing the hyperbaric chamber.

The air we breathe is composed of 21% oxygen, 78% of nitrogen, and 1% trace gases. Henry's law states that the amount of gas that dissolves in a liquid is proportional to the pressure exerted on the surface of the liquid. Therefore, as the partial pressure of the gas above a liquid increases, the amount of that gas that dissolves in the liquid also increases. HBO capitalizes upon Henry's Law by significantly increasing the ambient Po_2, causing a dramatic increase in the amount of dissolved oxygen carried by the blood. As the partial pressure of oxygen reaches 100 mm Hg, hemoglobin becomes fully saturated.

The content of oxygen in the blood is equal to the oxygen carried by hemoglobin and the oxygen dissolved in the blood. Oxygen content = $(1.34 \times HgB \times \%Saturation) + (0.003 \times Pao_2)$ Under normobaric conditions, the dissolved oxygen is negligible, representing only 0.3 mL of oxygen per 100 mL of blood (called volume percent—vol%), compared with 20 vol% carried by hemoglobin. Under hyperbaric conditions however, the Pao_2 at 3.0 ATA is greater than 2200 mm Hg. This is high enough to generate 5.4 vol% of dissolved oxygen, which can sustain basal metabolic functions in the complete absence of any hemoglobin!

Abbreviations: HBO, hyperbaric oxygen; PaO_2, partial pressure of oxygen in arterial blood.
From Wheelan HT, Kindwall EP. Hyperbaric medicine practice. 4th edition. Flagstaff (AZ): Best Publishing Company; 2017.

present with normocytic normochromic anemia, which may be due to combination of anemias, such as microcytic and macrocytic anemia (IDA and vitamin B_{12} deficiency).[2,5,17,27] Ferritin is useful for further differentiation, as discussed.

PATIENT DISPOSITION

Patients with vital sign abnormalities owing to anemia, those who require transfusion, and those with ongoing bleeding that is significant may require hospital admission.[2,5,33,34] Comorbidities including older age, congestive heart failure, and renal disease are also significant considerations in admission.[2,5,33,34] Hemodynamically stable patients with no active bleeding or ischemia may be discharged with follow-up, although consultation may be required depending on the specific bleeding site (GI, gynecology, etc). A clear follow-up plan with specific instructions is recommended.

REFERENCES

1. Irwin JJ, Kirchner JT. Anemia in children. Am Fam Physician 2001;64:1379–86.
2. Vieth JT, Lane DR. Anemia. Emerg Med Clin North Am 2014;32:613–28.
3. Rempher KJ, Little J. Assessment of red blood cell and coagulation laboratory data. AACN Clin Issues 2004;15(4):622–37.
4. World Health Organization (WHO). Haemoglobin concentrations for the diagnosis of anaemia and assessment of severity. Vitamin and Mineral Nutrition Information System. Geneva, World Health Organization, 2011 (WHO/NMH/NHD/MNM/11.1). Available at: http://www.who.int.vmnis/indicators/haemoglobin.pdf. Accessed October 19, 2017.
5. Bryan LJ, Zakai NA. Why is my patient anemic? Hematol Oncol Clin North Am 2012;26:205–30.
6. Marks PW. Approach to anemia in the adult and child. In: Hoffman R, Benz EJ, Silbersten LE, et al, editors. Hematology: basic principles and practice. 6th edition. Philadelphia: Elsevier; 2013.
7. McClean E, Cogswell M, Egli I, et al. Worldwide prevalence of anemia, WHO vitamin and mineral nutrition system, 1993-2005. Public Health Nutr 2009; 12(4):444–54.
8. Tettamanti M, Lucca U, Gandini F, et al. Prevalence, incidence and types of mild anemia in the elderly: the "Health and Anemia" population-based study. Haematologica 2010;95(11):1849–56.
9. McCormick L, Stott DJ. Anaemia in elderly patients. Clin Med 2007;7:501–4.
10. Beutler E, West C. Hematologic differences between African-Americans and whites: the roles of iron deficiency and alpha-thalassemia on hemoglobin levels and mean corpuscular volume. Blood 2005;106(2):740–5.
11. Dubois RW, Goodnough LT, Ershler WB, et al. Identification, diagnosis and management of anemia in adult ambulatory patients treated by primary care physicians: evidence-based and consensus recommendations. Curr Med Res Opin 2006;22(2):385–95.
12. Kaushansky K, Beutler E, Lichtman MA, et al, editors. Williams hematology. 8th edition. New York: McGraw-Hill Medical; 2011.
13. Janz TG, Hamilton GC. Anemia, polycythemia, and white blood cell disorders. In: Marx JA, Hockberger RS, Walls RM, et al, editors. Rosen's emergency medicine concepts and clinical practice. 7th edition. Philadelphia: Mosby Elsevier; 2010.
14. Quaglino D, Ginaldi L, Furia N, et al. The effect of age on hemostasis. Aging Clin Exp Res 1996;8:1–12.

15. Nissenson AR, Goodnough LT, Dubois RW. Anemia: not just an innocent bystander? Arch Intern Med 2003;163(12):1400–4.
16. Balducci L. Epidemiology of anemia in the elderly: information on diagnostic evaluation. J Am Geriatr Soc 2003;51:S2–9.
17. Ania BJ, Suman VJ, Fairbanks VF, et al. Prevalence of anemia in medical practice community versus referral patients. Mayo Clin Proc 1994;69(8):730–5.
18. Lee AI, Okam MM. Anemia in pregnancy. Hematol Oncol Clin North Am 2011; 25:241–59.
19. Hvas A, Nexo E. Diagnosis and treatment of vitamin B12 deficiency. An update. Haematologica 2006;91:1506–12.
20. Dharmarajan TS. Anemia in the long-term setting: routine screening and differential diagnosis. Consult Pharm 2008;23(Suppl A):5–10.
21. Woodman R, Ferrucci L, Guralnik J. Anemia in older adults. Curr Opin Hematol 2005;12:123–8.
22. Lipschitz D. Medical and functional consequences of anemia in the elderly. J Am Geriatr Soc 2003;51(Suppl):S10–3.
23. Steensma DP, Tefferi A. Anemia in the elderly: how should we define it, when does it matter, and what can be done? Mayo Clin Proc 2007;82(8):958–66.
24. Koury MJ. Abnormal erythropoiesis and the pathophysiology of chronic anemia. Blood Rev 2014;28(2):49–66.
25. deBack DJ, Kostova EB, van Kraaij M, et al. Of macrophages and red blood cells; a complex love story. Front Physiol 2014;5:9.
26. Spivak J. Prediction of chemotherapy-induced anaemia: is knowledge really power? Lancet Oncol 2005;6(11):822–4.
27. Smith DL. Anemia in the elderly. Am Fam Physician 2000;62(7):1565–72.
28. Scott RB. Common blood disorders: a primary care approach. Geriatrics 1993; 48(4):72–6, 79–80.
29. Baron BJ, Scalea TM. Acute blood loss. Emerg Med Clin North Am 1996;14(1): 35–56.
30. Hebert PC, Van der Linden P, Biro G, et al. Physiologic aspects of anemia. Crit Care Clin 2004;20:187–212.
31. Weiskopf R, Viele MK, Feiner J, et al. Human cardiovascular and metabolic response to acute, severe isovolemic anemia. JAMA 1998;279(3):217–21.
32. Robertson JJ, Brem E, Koyfman A. The acute hemolytic anemias: the importance of emergency diagnosis and management. J Emerg Med 2017;53(2): 202–11.
33. Carson JL, Guyatt G, Heddle NM, et al. Clinical practice guidelines from the AABB red blood cell transfusion thresholds and storage. JAMA 2016;316(19): 2025–35.
34. Long B, Koyfman A. Red blood cell transfusion in the emergency department. J Emerg Med 2016;51(2):120–30.
35. Huffstutler SY. Adult anemia. Adv Nurse Pract 2000;8:89–91.
36. Harder L, Boshkov L. The optimal hematocrit. Crit Care Clin 2010;26:335–54.
37. Finch CA, Lenfant C. Oxygen transport in man. N Engl J Med 1972;286:407–15.
38. Hameed SM, Aird WC. Oxygen delivery. Crit Care Med 2003;31:S658–67.
39. Dhaliwal G, Cornett PA, Tierney LM. Hemolytic anemia. Am Fam Physician 2004; 69(11):2599–606.
40. Myers MW. Antihypertensive drugs and the risk of idiopathic aplastic anemia. Br J Clin Pharmacol 2000;49(6):604–8.
41. Lubran MM. Hematologic side effects of drugs. Ann Clin Lab Sci 1989;19(2): 114–21.

42. Vandendries ER, Drews RE. Drug-associated disease: hematologic dysfunction. Crit Care Clin 2006;22:347–55.
43. Klein HG, Spahn DR, et al. Red blood cell transfusion in clinical practice. Lancet 2007;370:415–26.
44. Tefferi A. Anemia in adults: a contemporary approach to diagnosis. Mayo Clin Proc 2003;78:1274–80.
45. Chernecky CC, Berger BJ, editors. Laboratory tests and diagnostic procedures. 6th edition. St Louis (MO): Saunders; 2013.
46. Drews RE. Critical issues in hematology: anemia, thrombocytopenia, coagulopathy, and blood product transfusions in critically ill patients. Clin Chest Med 2003;24:607–22.
47. Gupta S, Ahern K, Nakhl F, et al. Clinical usefulness of haptoglobin levels to evaluate hemolysis in recently transfused patients. Adv Hematol 2011;2011:1–4.
48. Aslinia F, Mazza JJ, Yale SH. Megaloblastic anemia and other causes of macrocytosis. Clin Med Res 2006;4(3):236–41.
49. Beyer I, Compte N, Busuioc A, et al. Anemia and transfusions in geriatric patients: a time for evaluation. Hematology 2010;15(2):116–21.
50. Holcomb JB, del Junco DJ, Fox EE, et al, PROMMTT Study Group. The Prospective, Observational, Multicenter, Major Trauma Transfusion (PROMMTT) study: comparative effectiveness of a time-varying treatment with competing risks. JAMA Surg 2013;148(2):127–36.
51. Holcomb JB, Tilley BC, Baraniuk S. Transfusion of plasma, platelets, and red blood cells in a 1:1:1 vs a 1:1:2 ratio and mortality in patients with severe trauma. The PROPPR randomized clinical trial. JAMA 2015;313(5):471–82.
52. World Health Organization (WHO). Blood safety and availability. Available at: http://www.who.int/mediacentre/factsheets/fs279/en/. Accessed January 25, 2016.
53. Whitaker BI, Rajbhandary S, Harris A. The 2013 AABB blood collection, utilization, and patient blood management survey report. Bethesda (MD): AABB; 2015.
54. US Department of Health and Human Services. The 2009 national blood collection and utilization survey report. Washington, DC: US Department of Health and Human Services, Office of the Assistant Secretary for Health; 2011.
55. Takei T, Amin NA, Schmid G, et al. Progress in global blood safety for HIV. J Acquir Immune Defic Syndr 2009;52(suppl 2):S127–31.
56. Vincent JL, Baron JF, Reinhart K, et al. Anemia and blood transfusion in critically ill patients. JAMA 2002;288:1499–507.
57. Blood Observational Study Investigators of ANZICS-Clinical Trials Group, Westbrook A, Pettila V, Nichol A, et al. Transfusion practice and guidelines in Australian and New Zealand intensive care units. Intensive Care Med 2010; 36:1138–46.
58. Liumbruno G, Bennardello F, Lattanzio A, et al. Recommendations for the transfusion of red blood cells. Blood Transfus 2009;7:49–64.
59. National Health and Medical Research Council, Australian Government website. Clinical practice guidelines on the use of blood components (red blood cells, platelets, fresh frozen plasma, cryoprecipitate). Available at: http://www.nhmrc.gov.au/_files_nhmrc/publications/attachments/cp78_cp_blood_components.pdf. Accessed August 29, 2017.
60. American Red Cross website. Practice guidelines for blood transfusion: a compilation from recent peer-reviewed literature. Available at: http://chapters.

redcross.org/br/indianaoh/hospitals/transfusionguidelines.htm.re. Accessed August 29, 2017.
61. Elzik ME, Dirschl DR, Dahners LE. Correlation of transfusion volume to change in hematocrit. Am J Hematol 2006;81:145–6.
62. Adams RC, Lundy JS. Anesthesia in cases of poor surgical risk: some suggestions for decreasing the risk. Surg Gynecol Obstet 1942;74:10–1.
63. Wang JK, Klein HG. Red blood cell transfusion in the treatment and management of anaemia: the search for the elusive transfusion trigger. Vox Sang 2010;98:2–11.
64. Fakhry SM, Fata P. How low is too low? Cardiac risks with anemia. Crit Care 2004;8(Suppl 2):S11–4.
65. Hebert PC, Wells G, Blajchman MA, et al. A multicenter, randomized, controlled clinical trial of transfusion requirements in critical care. Transfusion requirements in critical care investigators, Canadian critical care trials group. N Engl J Med 1999;340:409–17.
66. Carson JL, Carless PA, Hebert PC. Transfusion thresholds and other strategies for guiding allogeneic red blood cell transfusion. Cochrane Database Syst Rev 2012;(4):CD002042.
67. Carless PA, Henry DA, Carson JL, et al. Transfusion thresholds and other strategies for guiding allogeneic red blood cell transfusion. Cochrane Database Syst Rev 2010;(10):CD002042.
68. Salpeter SR, Buckley JS, Chatterjee S. Impact of more restrictive blood transfusion strategies on clinical outcomes: a meta-analysis and systematic review. Am J Med 2014;127:124–31.e3.
69. Holst LB, Petersen MW, Haase N, et al. Restrictive versus liberal transfusion strategy for red blood cell transfusion: systematic review of randomised trials with meta-analysis and trial sequential analysis. BMJ 2015;350:h1354.
70. Holst LB, Haase N, Wetterslev J, et al. Lower versus higher hemoglobin threshold for transfusion in septic shock. N Engl J Med 2014;371:1381–91.
71. The ProCESS Investigators, Yealy DM, Kellum JA, Huang DT, et al. A randomized trial of protocol-based care for early septic shock. N Engl J Med 2014;370:1683–93.
72. The ARISE Investigators, ANZICS Clinical Trials Group, Peake SL, Delaney A, Bailey M. Goal-directed resuscitation for patients with early septic shock. N Engl J Med 2014;371:1496–506.
73. Villanueva C, Colomo A, Bosch A, et al. Transfusion strategies for acute upper gastrointestinal bleeding. N Engl J Med 2013;368:11–21.
74. Restellini S, Kherad O, Jairath V, et al. Red blood cell transfusion is associated with increased rebleeding in patients with nonvariceal upper gastrointestinal bleeding. Aliment Pharmacol Ther 2013;37:316–22.
75. Jairath V, Kahan BC, Gray A, et al. Restrictive versus liberal blood transfusion for acute upper gastrointestinal bleeding (TRIGGER): a pragmatic, open-label, cluster randomised feasibility trial. Lancet 2015;386:137–44.
76. Baraniuk S, Tilley BC, del Junco DJ, et al. Pragmatic Randomized Optimal Platelet and Plasma Ratios (PROPPR) trial: design, rationale and implementation. Injury 2014;45:1287–95.
77. McIntyre L, Hebert PC, Wells G, et al. Is a restrictive transfusion strategy safe for resuscitated and critically ill trauma patients? J Trauma 2004;57:563–8.
78. Brakenridge SC, Phelan HA, Henley SS, et al. Early blood product and crystalloid volume resuscitation: risk association with multiple organ dysfunction after severe blunt traumatic injury. J Trauma 2011;71:299–305.

79. Johnson JL, Moore EE, Kashuk JL, et al. Effect of blood products transfusion on the development of postinjury multiple organ failure. Arch Surg 2010;145:973–7.

80. Bochicchio GV, Napolitano L, Joshi M, et al. Outcome analysis of blood product transfusion in trauma patients: a prospective, risk adjusted study. World J Surg 2008;32:2185–9.

81. Levy PS, Kim SJ, Eckel PK, et al. Limit to cardiac compensation during acute isovolemic hemodilution: influence of coronary stenosis. Am J Physiol 1993; 265:H340–9.

82. Sabatine MS, Morrow DA, Giugliano RP, et al. Association of hemoglobin levels with clinical outcomes in acute coronary syndromes. Circulation 2005;111: 2042–9.

83. Ripolles Melchor J, Casans Frances R, Espinosa A, et al. Restrictive versus liberal transfusion strategy for red blood cell transfusion in critically ill patients and in patients with acute coronary syndrome: a systematic review, meta-analysis and trial sequential analysis. Minerva Anestesiol 2016;82(5):582–98.

84. Rao SV, Jollis JG, Harrington RA, et al. Relationship of blood transfusion and clinical outcomes in patients with acute coronary syndromes. JAMA 2004;292: 1555–62.

85. Chatterjee S, Wetterslev J, Sharma A, et al. Association of blood transfusion with increased mortality in myocardial infarction: a meta-analysis and diversity-adjusted study sequential analysis. JAMA Intern Med 2013;173:132–9.

86. LeRoux P. Haemoglobin management in acute brain injury. Curr Opin Crit Care 2013;19:83–91.

87. Diedler J, Sykora M, Hahn P, et al. Low hemoglobin is associated with poor functional outcome after non-traumatic, supratentorial intracerebral hemorrhage. Crit Care 2010;14:R63.

88. Oddo M, Milby A, Chen I, et al. Hemoglobin concentration and cerebral metabolism in patients with aneurysmal subarachnoid hemorrhage. Stroke 2009; 40:1275–81.

89. McIntyre LA, Fergusson DA, Hutchison JS, et al. Effect of a liberal versus restrictive transfusion strategy on mortality in patients with moderate to severe head injury. Neurocrit Care 2006;5:4–9.

90. Boutin A, Chasse M, Shemilt M, et al. Red blood cell transfusion in patients with traumatic brain injury: a systematic review and metaanalysis. Transfus Med Rev 2016;30:15–24.

91. Federowicz I, Barrett BB, Andersen JW, et al. Characterization of reactions after transfusion of cellular blood components that are white cell reduced before storage. Transfusion 1996;36(1):21–8.

92. Popovsky MA, Audet AM, Andrzejewski C Jr. Transfusion-associated circulatory overload in orthopedic surgery patients: a multi-institutional study. Immunohematology 1996;12(2):87–9.

93. Clifford L, Jia Q, Yadav H, et al. Characterizing the epidemiology of perioperative transfusion-associated circulatory overload. Anesthesiology 2015;122(1): 21–8.

94. DeBaun MR, Gordon M, McKinstry RC, et al. Controlled trial of transfusions for silent cerebral infarcts in sickle cell anemia. N Engl J Med 2014;371(8):699–710.

95. Sanguis Study Group. Use of blood products for elective surgery in 43 European hospitals. Transfus Med 1994;4(4):251–68.

96. Zou S, Dorsey KA, Notari EP, et al. Prevalence, incidence, and residual risk of human immunodeficiency virus and hepatitis C virus infections among United

States blood donors since the introduction of nucleic acid testing. Transfusion 2010;50(7):1495–504.

97. Stramer SL, Notari EP, Krysztof DE, et al. Hepatitis B virus testing by minipool nucleic acid testing: does it improve blood safety? Transfusion 2013;53(10 pt 2):2449–58.

98. US Food and Drug Administration. Transfusion/donation fatalities: notification process for transfusion related fatalities and donation related deaths. Available at: http://www.fda.gov/BiologicsBloodVaccines/SafetyAvailability/ReportaProblem/TransfusionDonationFatalities/. Accessed August 1, 2017.

99. Clark S. Iron deficiency anemia: diagnosis and management. Curr Opin Gastroenterol 2009;25:122–9.

100. Weiss G, Gordeuk VR. Benefits and risks of iron therapy for chronic anaemias. Eur J Clin Invest 2005;35(Suppl 3):36–45.

101. Helman A. Episode 65 – IV Iron for anemia in emergency medicine. Emergency medicine cases. 2015. Available at: https://emergencymedicinecases.com/iv-iron-for-anemia-in-emergency-medicine/. Accessed October 15, 2017.

102. Cançado RD, Muñoz M. Intravenous iron therapy: how far have we come? Rev Bras Hematol Hemoter 2011;33(6):461–9.

103. Damon L. Anemias of chronic disease in the aged: diagnosis and treatment. Geriatrics 1992;47:47–57.

104. Litton E, Xiao J, Ho KM. Safety and efficacy of intravenous iron therapy in reducing requirement for allogeneic blood transfusion: systematic review and meta-analysis of randomised clinical trials. BMJ 2013;347:f4822.

105. Munoz M, Gómez-Ramírez S, Cuenca J, et al. Very-short-term perioperative intravenous iron administration and postoperative outcome in major orthopedic surgery: a pooled analysis of observational data from 2547 patients. Transfusion 2014;54(2):289–99.

106. Van Meter KW. Undersea and hyperbaric oxygen medical society. Severe anemia. Hyperbaric oxygen therapy indications. p. 209–13.

107. Van Meter KW. A systematic review of the literature reporting the application of hyperbaric oxygen in the treatment of exceptional blood loss anemia: an evidence-based approach. Undersea Hyperb Med 2005;32(1):61–83.

108. Barton S, editor. Clinical evidence. London: BMJ Publishing Group; 2001.

109. Bitterman H, Reissman P, Bitterman N, et al. Oxygen therapy in hemorrhagic shock. Circ Shock 1991;33:183–91.

110. Pediatric nutrition handbook. 6th edition. Elk Grove Village (IL): American Academy of Pediatrics; 2009. p. 403–22.

111. U.S. Preventive Services Task Force. Screening for iron deficiency anemia including iron supplementation for children and pregnancy women: Recommendation Statement. Publication No. AHRQ 06–0589, May 2006.

112. Kohli-Kumar M. Screening for anemia in children: AAP recommendations- a critique. Pediatrics 2001;108:E56.

113. American Society of Anesthesiologists Task Force on Perioperative Blood Management. Practice guidelines for perioperative blood management: an updated report by the American Society of Anesthesiologists Task Force on Perioperative Blood Management*. Anesthesiology 2015;122(2):241–75.

114. Janus J, Moerschel SK. Evaluation of anemia in children. Am Fam Physician 2010;81(12):1462–71.

115. Kristinsson G, Shtivelman S, Hom J, et al. Prevalence of occult anemia in an urban pediatric emergency department: what is our response? Pediatr Emerg Care 2012;28(4):313–5.

116. Salive ME, Cornoni-Huntley J, Guralnik JM, et al. Anemia and hemoglobin levels in older persons: relationship with age, gender, and health status. J Am Geriatr Soc 1992;40:489–96.
117. Daly MP. Anemia in the elderly. Am Fam Physician 1989;39:129–36.
118. Elis A, Ravid M, Manor Y, et al. A clinical approach to 'idiopathic' normocytic-normochromic anemia? J Am Geriatr Soc 1996;44:832–4.
119. Seward SJ, Safran C, Marton KI, et al. Does the mean corpuscular volume help physicians evaluate hospitalized patients with anemia? J Gen Intern Med 1990; 5:187–91.
120. Lipschitz DA. The anemia of chronic disease. J Am Geriatr Soc 1990;38: 1258–64.
121. Cash JM, Sears DA. The anemia of chronic disease: spectrum of associated diseases in a series of unselected hospitalized patients. Am J Med 1989;87: 638–44.
122. Kent S, Weinberg ED, Stuart-Macadam P. The etiology of the anemia of chronic disease and infection. J Clin Epidemiol 1994;47:23–33.
123. Walsh JR. Hematologic problems. In: Cassel CK, et al, editors. Geriatric medicine. New York: Springer; 1997. p. 627–36.

The Cancer Emergency Department—The Ohio State University James Cancer Center Experience

Luca R. Delatore, MD

KEYWORDS

- Oncology emergency department • Emergency oncology • Hematology
- Administration

KEY POINTS

- Extensive prior planning is necessary to create a fully integrated cancer emergency department that interfaces seamlessly with the rest of the hospital system.
- Significant emphasis must be placed on building relationships between experts across disciplines in emergency medicine and hematology or oncology.
- Using providers who are cross-trained in hematology or oncology and emergency medicine makes the safest and most effective care team.
- Ongoing adjustments of resources are important to provide the safest and most effective model for emergency cancer care.

In 2014, there were an estimated 14.7 million people in the United States with cancer.[1] The rate of cancer diagnosis has been increasing over the last 20 years. In 2017, it is projected that 1.7 million more cases will be diagnosed with 67% surviving for at least 5 years postdiagnosis.[1,2] As this population increases, the need for continued access to quality emergency care will likewise grow.

Patients with cancer account for 4.2% of all emergency department (ED) visits in the United States with an admission rate of 59%.[3] These patients are typically seen for not only cancer-related problems (eg, infection, local mass effect, pleural effusions, ascites, side-effects of chemotherapy, and hematologic and metabolic problems), they can also present for any other noncancer-related emergency.[4-7] As such, there is a significant need for EDs that can care for this unique population.

In 2010, The University of Texas MD Anderson Cancer Center created the first cancer ED within a comprehensive cancer center. In 2015, The James Cancer Hospital's ED (JED) opened as an integrated portion of The Ohio State University Wexner

Disclosure Statement: None.
Department of Emergency Medicine, Emergency Services, Wexner Medical Center at The Ohio State University, 760 Prior Hall, 410 West 10th Avenue, Columbus, OH 43210, USA
E-mail address: Luca.delatore@osumc.edu

Emerg Med Clin N Am 36 (2018) 631–636
https://doi.org/10.1016/j.emc.2018.04.012
0733-8627/18/© 2018 Elsevier Inc. All rights reserved.

Medical Center's ED (OSUED). This was the first cancer ED that was fully integrated into a larger and comprehensive ED.

THE DESIGN PHASE

The initial planning, which began in 2012, was multidisciplinary and studied multiple areas of patient care. This included patient simulations and provider and patient panels. The major areas to be considered were hours of operation, staff education, and work flow studies. A retrospective quantitative analysis of patients with an oncology diagnosis presenting to the ED was performed using electronic medical records to confirm the concept, as well as predict volume and acuity. The review assessed and projected trends in chief complaints, primary oncology diagnoses, arrival day of week, time of day, mode, patient acuity, and ED length of stay.

During the early design phase of The James Cancer Hospital's Cancer and Critical Care Tower, a decision was made to expand the OSUED to include a designated treatment area for oncology and hematology patients. The original plans, drafted in 2006, set forward the intention to relocate The James Cancer Hospital's ambulatory Immediate Care Center into the expanding ED. As construction of the building developed, the expected growth in the oncology population, patient acuity, and complexities related to the disease continuum were key factors that eventually drove the innovative concept of creating a fully integrated ED for hematologic and oncologic emergencies. Throughout the planning phases, patient input and system priorities were identified, and strategies were designed and tested to improve workflow, create efficiencies, improve patient throughput, and develop an elite patient experience.

Significant emphasis was placed on building relationships between experts and across disciplines in emergency medicine, hematology, and oncology. Before opening, multiple 3-day intensive planning retreats were held to ensure key stakeholders were involved in the decision-making process. A substantial amount of time was dedicated to develop and analyze how success would be measured, and what needed to be done to appropriately manage oncologic emergencies in a new environment. The time to plan and provide constant communication on progress was critical to the successful launch of the first fully integrated, ED focused on hematology and oncology in a brand new 1.1 million square foot, 306 inpatient bed, cancer hospital. Another critical aspect of the preparation involved education provided to outpatient oncology and hematology clinics. Informational presentations allowed for staff education and clinical feedback, and, ultimately, set expectations. A multidisciplinary case–based conference was developed to help with education of the staff. The monthly conference offers continued education opportunities and has been used to present interesting cases, new therapy options, and best practice paradigms.

THE PHYSICAL SPACE

Fifteen of the 106 ED treatment spaces were designated for cancer-related emergencies and carefully designed with the specialized population in mind. The rooms were designed to be flexible to accommodate both patients with cancer and patients without cancer when necessary. An internal waiting area for patients with the potential for immunosuppression was created and private restrooms were factored into the design. A room was also designated adjacent to the internal waiting room to allow for initial patient treatment in a private area if no rooms were available to place the patient. The design of the internal waiting room was also intentional, with special attention paid to create a quiet and soothing environment.

The unit consists of 5 treatment areas with recliners for low-to-moderate acuity patients to receive rapid evaluation and treatment, as well as 10 traditional, private, monitored examination and/or treatment rooms. One room is equipped to care for patients who require negative airflow and 7 are designed with private restrooms.

The decision was made to centralize the care team, placing the physician, advanced practice provider (APP), and charge nurse in a contiguous area. This was important to ensure efficiency, improve patient flow, and multidisciplinary communication. Primary nurses, patient care associates, pharmacists, respiratory therapists, clerical support staff, and social service colleagues were also strategically placed near the core of the unit.

THE FLOW

Oncology-focused questions were built into the triage screening process to properly identify patients with cancer presenting to the ED in need of emergent care. The ED maintains a single entry into the facility. Patients are triaged in the traditional triage area, at bedside, or in the JED. Bedside registration is considered best practice in the JED when possible. The incidence and prevalence of urgent or emergent oncologic and hematologic conditions were tracked and researched during design. Initial areas of opportunity included recognition and treatment of chemotherapy-induced side-effects, fever in the patient with cancer, and pain in patients with acute vasoocclusive crisis related to sickle cell disease. Triage protocols and individualized treatment plans were developed in the electronic medical record to guide evidence-informed care. Guidelines for treatment of common oncologic emergencies, including metabolic or endocrinal, hematologic, and structural, were developed and imbedded into training for all clinical staff and providers.

THE PROVIDERS AND STAFF

Provider staffing for the specialized section of the JED includes attending physicians, APPs, and resident physicians. Emphasis was placed on hiring staff with experience or interest in care of the oncology patient. The APPs were chosen for their previous expertise in emergency medicine or oncology and were extensively trained in whichever component they did not originally have experience with. Treating the oncology patient is complex and the decision was made to dedicate not only APPs but also physician providers to the JED with the aim of having a core group of consistent providers. Dedicated attending physician coverage totals 12 hours per day, with the remainder of the day being covered by attendings from the main OSUED.

As with any major teaching hospital, resident physician coverage is important for patient care. The acuity of the patients in the JED represents a unique opportunity for learning and procedural mastery. The most common procedures performed are airway management, central access, bedside ultrasound, thoracentesis, and paracentesis. The high concentration of hematology and oncology patients ensures that resident physicians are able to care for critically ill patients. The area also has a dedicated shift for medical students rotating in the OSUED. The decision was also made to start a 1-year non-accreditation council for graduate medical education (ACGME) fellowship designed to give graduates the chance to focus on the JED, inpatient oncology, and hematology services.

Nursing staff from the cancer program with significant training in hematology, oncology, bone marrow transplant, and/or critical care were provided rigorous personalized emergency medicine education and orientation. Another key aspect of the care team is dedicated case managers and social services. Beyond the complexity of their medical illness, many patients have complex social concerns that are related to their presentation. Having these services available in the JED allows for early intervention with the patients and family.

THE EXPERIENCE

Since the JED opened in April 2015, patterns have developed in types of patients presenting for treatment, as well as in acuity. Most patients present for cancer-related presentations. Symptom control related to the primary diagnosis or cancer treatment is the most common reason for presentation. There are a significant number of patients transferred from outside medical facilities for cancer care. The geographic distribution of the patients transferred to the JED includes not only patients from local hospitals in central Ohio but also from as far away as West Virginia and Kentucky. Many patients with cancer present to the JED for routine care that may not require specialized cancer care because they have grown comfortable with the level of care and familiarity with their disease that the JED providers can offer.

The overall admission rate has consistently been high, ranging from 60% to 65% of all patients seen. This does not seem to be skewed by presentation to the JED because review of admissions shows most meet inpatient criteria versus observation status. The patients are assigned an Emergency Severity Index (ESI) score based on a triage algorithm that provides clinically relevant stratification of patients into 5 groups from 1 (most urgent) to 5 (least urgent). This acuity score seems to correlate to admission rate, with more than 50% of patients assigned an ESI score of 1 or 2. Only 1% of the patients seen in the JED have an ESI of 5. There has also been a consistent growth trend at the JED. Since opening, the number of new patients to the Ohio State University Wexner Medical Center system and The James Comprehensive Cancer Center is 1.0 to 1.5 per day. This has created some difficulty establishing prompt follow-up for new patients.

After experiencing higher than expected acuity, volume, and admission rates, the decision was made to transform the original 5 recliner treatment spaces into monitored treatment spaces. This allowed for these 5 treatment spaces to remain open for longer periods of time and monitor a higher acuity patient. The time trends of ED arrival have also been tracked. This allows for adaptation of the provider coverage schedule and helps with patient flow. Slightly greater than 45% of the patients present between 11 AM and 7 PM, and another 20% of patients present between 7 PM and 11 PM In contrast, less than 10% of patients present during the early morning hours of 3 to 7 AM. Monday and Tuesday were also found to be the most common days for presentation. The top admission diagnoses include abdominal pain, shortness of breath, fever, sickle cell crisis, chest pain, vomiting, altered mental status, headache, chest pain, critical laboratory values, and back pain.

Since opening the JED in April of 2015, the most common cancer diagnoses were tracked and placed into disease groups to compare with preopening data from 2014. The most common presentations have been related to gastrointestinal cancer (15%), sickle cell disease (14%), and lung cancer (12%). Evaluation for cancers of the breast, lymphoma, or leukemia, central nervous system disease, gynecologic, urologic, and head or neck cancer all ranged from 4% to 6% of total patients seen. The number of patients presenting for sickle cell complications decreased in 2017 secondary to the opening of the Sickle Cell Day Hospital (SCDH) in an area separate from the JED. The unit has been able to provide treatment of sickle cell patients on a daily basis and prevent readmission to the hospital. Patients can schedule appointments for the SCDH. If the APP in the SCDH feels that patient is too acute for treatment, the patient is transported to the JED for registration and evaluation. Conversely, if patients arrive at the JED and do not need emergent treatment, they can be screened by the APP and transported to the SCDH if beds are available.

The dedicated area in the ED allows for protocol development and process improvement specific to oncologic and hematologic emergencies. The initial areas of focus were either high-risk presentations or common complaints. Multidisciplinary teams were formed to study sepsis, febrile neutropenia, pain control, high utilizers, and sickle cell crisis. With a platform to improve patient care and the ability to further develop oncologic and hematologic emergency interventions came the opportunity to improve processes for patients with emergencies ranging from febrile neutropenia to pain management during acute sickle cell crisis. Multidisciplinary teams, including key clinicians from subspecialties, collaborated to address the need for improvement in 2 of the top JED utilizers, based on admitting diagnosis and chief complaint.

Ongoing management of emergency services for hematologic and oncologic patients plays a critical part in the success of a fully integrated ED, including encounter volume, patient placements, and quality metrics. The greatest challenges include intermittent inpatient capacity challenges and service line capitations, leading to increased boarding hours and limitation of treatment spaces for new patients.

THE PATIENT'S EXPERIENCE

Guiding principles during design and implementation included commitments to provide hematology and oncology patients with an exceptional ED experience in a care area that was tailored to their individualized needs and by staff with expert training in urgent or emergent management of their disease and its related complications. To measure the success of implementation, The James Cancer Hospital in collaboration with Press Ganey launched an ED patient satisfaction survey for discharged patients from the JED. The subset of patients is filtered from the OSUED and validated through a rigorous selection process. The patient satisfaction scores from the JED have consistently been higher than scores from the OSUED. A program was initiated in 2016 to call back the hematology and oncology patients who were discharged on the preceding day. Objectives for the call back program include follow-up on symptom management, experience, and continuity of care. Although results were positive, the program was discontinued secondary to staff availability. The long-term goal is to reimplement this process when resources are available. There was also coordination with an in-house nurse call line for patients of The James Comprehensive Cancer Center. In the past, this was outsourced and quality and results were varied. Successful implementation of this ongoing program decreased the number of unexpected presentations to the JED.

SUMMARY

As the first fully integrated oncology and hematology ED in the country, The James ED's integrated model has the potential to revolutionize the concept of oncologic emergency management. The opening of The James Comprehensive Cancer Center allowed the opportunity to improve the care of patients with oncologic and hematologic emergencies. Creating an integrated oncologic ED at a tertiary care hospital involves multidisciplinary planning and thoughtful preparation. The effect on outcomes such as time-sensitive care, ED length of stay, and patient satisfaction seem to be very positive, supporting the case that this model can serve as a blueprint for other tertiary care centers with high volumes of hematologic and oncologic patients requiring emergency care.

REFERENCES

1. Howlader N, Noone A, Krapcho M, et al. SEER cancer statistics review. 2017. Available at: https://seer.cancer.gov/csr/1975_2014/. Accessed October 27, 2017.
2. Bluethmann SM, Mariotto AB, Rowland JH. Anticipating the "silver tsunami": prevalence trajectories and comorbidity burden among older cancer survivors in the United States. Cancer Epidemiol Biomarkers Prev 2016;25(7):1029–36.
3. Rivera DR, Gallicchio L, Brown J, et al. Trends in adult cancer-related emergency department utilization: an analysis of data from the nationwide emergency department sample. JAMA Oncol 2017;3(10):e172450.
4. Wagner J, Arora S. Oncologic metabolic emergencies. Emerg Med Clin North Am 2014;32(3):509–25.
5. Khan UA, Shanholtz CB, McCurdy MT. Oncologic mechanical emergencies. Emerg Med Clin North Am 2014;32(3):495–508.
6. White L, Ybarra M. Neutropenic fever. Emerg Med Clin North Am 2014;32(3):549–61.
7. Young JS, Simmons JW. Chemotherapeutic medications and their emergent complications. Emerg Med Clin North Am 2014;32(3):563–78.

The Oncologic Emergency Medicine Fellowship

Michael G. Purcell, MD[a],*, Imad El Majzoub, MD[b]

KEYWORDS

- Oncologic emergency medicine • Fellowship • Cancer population
- Comprehensive cancer care

KEY POINTS

- Oncologic emergency medicine is a developing field in the United States that will require increasing attention as the population with cancer grows.
- The population with cancer in the emergency department is a specific subpopulation that encounters a variety of medical problems not normally seen in the noncancer population.
- An ideal oncologic emergency medicine fellowship would give attention to the comprehensive set of issues in cancer care, including emergent medical needs, palliative care, developing goals of care, and understanding of the psychosocial issues in cancer care.
- Currently, 2 models for the oncologic emergency medicine fellowship exist. One is located at The Ohio State University and the other at MD Anderson.

BACKGROUND

Over the past 20 years, the prevalence of cancer has been increasing in the United States. In 2014, there were an estimated 14.7 million Americans living with a cancer diagnosis.[1] There were an estimated 1,7 million additional people diagnosed with some form of malignancy in 2017. This number is expected to stay the same in 2018.[1] Of these patients, 67% are estimated to survive at least 5 years following their diagnosis.[1] Barring any miraculous paradigm shifts in cancer treatments, by 2040, there will be an estimated 26 million patients with active cancer or who have previously had cancer, 73% of whom are projected to be older than the age of 65 years.[2] As this patient population grows and ages, it will need to have continued access to quality emergency care before, during, and following treatment of their malignancy.

Recent trends in this growing population have shown that patients with a cancer diagnosis account for 4.2% of all emergency department visits in the United States.[3] These visits include evaluation for infection, emergencies related to the malignancy,

Disclosure Statement: The authors have no financial disclosures.
[a] Department of Emergency Medicine, The Ohio State University, 750 Prior Hall, 376 West 10th Avenue, Columbus, OH 43210, USA; [b] Department of Emergency Medicine, UT MD Anderson Cancer Center, 1515 Holcombe boulevard, Unit 1468, Houston, TX 77030, USA
* Corresponding author.
E-mail address: Michael.Purcell@osumc.edu

Emerg Med Clin N Am 36 (2018) 637–643
https://doi.org/10.1016/j.emc.2018.04.013
0733-8627/18/© 2018 Elsevier Inc. All rights reserved.

emed.theclinics.com

and treatment side-effects, as well as the entire spectrum of nononcologic emergencies. After emergency department evaluation, 59% of these patients were ultimately admitted to the hospital compared with 16% of patients without a cancer diagnosis.[3]

Patients with cancer represent a unique population in emergency medicine. These patients constitute a significant portion of emergency department visits and have a high rate of admission.[3] In addition, they are at increased risk of developing life-threatening emergencies not routinely seen in patients without cancer.[4–7] Such emergencies can be a result of the malignancy itself because it poses the risk of metastases, local mass effect, local tissue invasion, and hematologic and metabolic derangements.[4,5] Alternatively, the emergencies may be related to treatment of the malignancy because these patients are subject to aggressive treatment regimens that carry a significant risk of adverse effects.[6,7] As this population continues to grow and seek access to emergent medical care, there is an increased need to evaluate, recognize, and treat the unique conditions inherent to the oncology patient, regardless of whether they are on active therapy or not. Given this growth, a need for increasing specialized care and knowledge of these patients is developing. Currently, 2 fellowship programs in emergency oncology exist at The Ohio State University and The University of Texas MD Anderson Cancer Center. These programs offer further advanced training within emergency oncology. The oncologic emergency medicine (OEM) fellows are in a unique position to evaluate, manage, and treat the undifferentiated patient with cancer. As emergency physicians, they are already trained in critical care and the initial diagnosis and management of surgical emergencies. Furthermore, they are trained in procedures, including intubation, paracentesis, thoracentesis, and lumbar puncture. This skill set allows for the rapid, efficient, and effective management of the undifferentiated patient who so often shows up in the emergency department.

THE IDEAL FELLOWSHIP EXPERIENCE

An OEM fellowship will enable emergency physicians to better deal with complications of patients with cancer presenting to emergency departments in terms of diagnosis, decision-making, and delivery of treatments. This helps to reduce mortality and morbidity, and provides patients with better standards of living after discharge. The ideal OEM fellowship should provide trainees with better understanding of all the aspects surrounding cancer care, including but not limited to prevention and acute and palliative care.[8]

The role of an emergency physician trained in OEM should not be limited to doing aggressive resuscitation and complicated procedures. It should also involve the primary and secondary prevention of cancer. Many cancer risk factors are addressed in the emergency medicine literature. These risk factors include but are not limited to carcinogenic viruses, tobacco use, alcohol abuse, and exposure to radiation.[9–12] Emergency physicians can orient their patients to do annual screenings for early detection of breast, cervical, and colorectal cancers.[13,14]

An OEM fellowship will enable the emergency physician to be knowledgeable about appropriate diagnostic and therapeutic approaches to patients with cancer who present to the emergency department for acute and emergent care.[15,16] An ideal fellowship program should allow the trainees to address acute oncologic care using a systematic approach via a thorough understanding of the nature and pathophysiology of the disease. This includes its complications related to disease progression, knowledge of the current cancer therapeutics and their side-effects, and the performance of complex procedures as a part of the acute care of patients with cancer. This approach is significantly different from that followed when dealing with patients without cancer.

Doctors should improve the quality of life for patients with cancer. An OEM fellowship should make the emergency physician aware of the prognosis of patients by addressing the course and the nature of the disease and goals of care while keeping in mind the overall prognosis for any given patient. A trainee should be able to discuss these issues freely with patients and the oncology partners involved in the patient's care. This will help to determine the magnitude of the treatment and can aid in improving the quality of end-of-life care.[17] Many studies stress the importance of initiating palliative care in the emergency department. This should drive a strong understanding and incorporation of palliative care as a main element in the curriculum of OEM fellowship programs.[18,19]

An ideal training program should not neglect the importance of research training for the trainees. This will help prepare fellows who want to pursue academic careers and to foster their ability to work in research-oriented institutions, especially in this era of new emerging cancer treatment modalities.[20] Trainees should be also able to participate in quality improvement projects to deliver the optimal care in a perfect environment for this delicate patient population.

THE CURRENT MODELS
The Ohio State University Wexner Medical Center

In 2014, the James Cancer Hospital at The Ohio State University Wexner Medical Center (OSUWMC) opened a 15-bed emergency department dedicated to the emergent care of patients with cancer. Although it functions as a separate treatment space, the James emergency department is fully integrated into the remainder of the OSUWMC emergency department and offers comprehensive care for its patients with cancer. Patients presenting to the James emergency department have access to the full cadre of specialists available at the OSUWMC. The James emergency department sees nearly 13,000 patients a year. Recognizing the need for further advanced care and education in this patient population, a fellowship in oncologic emergencies was recently developed. The fellowship was initiated in 2017. It is a 1-year fellowship with the mission of training emergency physicians in hematologic and oncologic emergencies. The goals of the OSUWMC fellowship are listed in **Box 1**.

The current OSUEM OEM fellowship is a 1-year program. It was developed as a multidisciplinary experience that involves

- 7 months of training in the James emergency department
- 1 month of training with the oncology service

Box 1
Goals of The Ohio State University Oncologic Emergency Fellowship

- Recognize and promptly manage the various hematologic and oncologic emergencies
- Develop an understanding of the role for pain and palliative medicine in the emergency department, including goals of care discussions
- Understand appropriate patient care in the emergency department, inpatient, and intensive care unit settings
- Be familiar with the various chemotherapies and management of their side effects
- Understand the side effects and management of radiation therapy
- Participate in a scholarly project of publishable quality
- Participate in quality improvement

- 1 month of training with the hematology service
- 1 month of training with the neurooncology service
- 1 month of training with the palliative medicine service
- 1 month of protected time for research.

The program is structured to expose the fellow to a variety of oncologic emergencies, malignancies, and treatment modalities. Additionally, the program seeks to expose the fellow to palliative care treatment of the patient with cancer.

The 1-month oncology rotation serves to expose the fellow to a variety of solid organ tumors and their treatments. The immersive experience is divided into 2 2-week blocks:

- During the first block, the fellow rotates on the oncology inpatient service. On this service, the fellow works with an attending oncologist and traditional hematology-oncology fellow to provide inpatient care in established patients with cancer. This includes management of the malignancy, treatment side-effects, and additional medical comorbidities. The need for procedural intervention, including paracentesis, thoracentesis, and lumbar puncture, is also addressed.
- The following 2 weeks are spent rotating with the oncology consult team. This team, composed of an oncologist and advanced practice providers, provides consultation services in the James Cancer Hospital and OSUWMC hospitals for patients with established cancer diagnoses or potential new cancer diagnoses. The consult team aids in workup of potential new cancers, staging of existing cancers, and guidance on continuation or withholding therapies in the setting of acute illness.

Similar to the oncology rotation, the hematology rotation is split into 2 blocks: 2 weeks are allotted to the inpatient team and 2 weeks to the consult team:

- On the inpatient team, the fellow works with an attending hematologist, as well as a traditional hematology-oncology fellow. The inpatient team cares for patients with established hematologic malignancy diagnoses. This includes chemotherapy, management of the malignancy, treatment side-effects, and additional medical comorbidities. These patients often need additional procedural intervention, most commonly lumbar puncture for administration of intrathecal chemotherapy and evaluation of metastatic burden.
- The hematology consult team is responsible for providing services in the James Cancer Hospital and OSUWMC hospitals. It is composed of an attending hematologist and a hematology-oncology fellow. The hematology consult team provides guidance on both malignant and benign hematology throughout the hospital system.

On the neurooncology rotation, the OEM fellow rotates with a James Cancer Hospital neurooncologist. The aim of this rotation is to improve knowledge of the management of primary brain tumors, metastatic disease, and leptomeningeal carcinomatosis. This experience aims to provide both inpatient and outpatient experience to help familiarize the fellow with the whole spectrum of severity in neurooncologic disease. The neurooncology team works closely with the works closely with the hematology, oncology, radiation and neurosurgery teams at the James Cancer Hospital to provide multidisciplinary care of their patients.

The palliative medicine rotation was incorporated into the fellowship as a means to improve symptom management in the emergency department. On this rotation, the fellow rotates with the palliative medicine team in the James Cancer Hospital. This team works with the inpatient services to provide patient-focused symptomatic treatment of cancer and treatment side-effects. This includes pain control, antiemetics for nausea and vomiting, and treatments for constipation and diarrhea, with the goal of improving patient quality of life.

The OSUOEM fellowship allocates a month for research and other scholarly activities. One expectation for graduation from the fellowship is completion of a scholarly activity that looks into an aspect of emergency cancer care. This block of time offers protected time away from both off-service rotations and emergency department shifts to allow for dedicated research. This time can be used to perform original research, prepare manuscripts for publication, prepare for presentations, and participate in quality improvement measures.

Although off-service rotations provide invaluable experience in the integrative and comprehensive care of the emergency oncology patient, the bulk of The Ohio State University fellowship program is rooted in the emergency department. Seven months are devoted to the James emergency department. During these months, the fellow works the bulk of their emergency department shifts in the James emergency department. The fellow functions as an emergency medicine attending who leads a team of advanced practice providers and emergency medicine residents in providing care for patients with cancer. This includes the manifestations of malignancy, treatment rendered for therapy side-effects, discussions on the goals of care, and management of additional emergent needs not related to the malignancy.

In addition to the defined curriculum, there is a significant amount of flexibility inherent to The Ohio State University OEM fellowship. This allows for each fellow to create his or her own niche in emergency oncology. The current model allows for a fellow to pursue administration, research, and education as their chosen path in this field. The Department of Emergency Medicine at The Ohio State University has significant representation in hospital administration, education, and research. This affords a fellow the opportunity to explore further interests within emergency oncology.

MD Anderson

In 2010, The University of Texas MD Anderson Cancer Center created the first academic department of emergency medicine within a comprehensive cancer center. The department of emergency medicine's mission is to provide efficient and timely care of the highest quality to those with cancer and to uphold MD Anderson's core value of caring, integrity, and discovery.

The OEM fellowship was established and approved in 2011 to provide training and insight into the emergency treatment of patients with cancer beyond that provided by traditional training programs in emergency medicine. This fellowship provides 12 to 24 months of advanced training in the growing subdiscipline of OEM. This 1-year (with an optional second year) fellowship offers an outstanding opportunity to highly qualified applicants who are interested in expanding their clinical knowledge in the areas of cancer-related emergencies, pain and symptom management, and palliative care.

At the completion of the first year, the fellow is expected to be knowledgeable about appropriate diagnostic and therapeutic approaches to patients with cancer who present to emergency department for acute care. Goals of the program are listed in **Box 2**.

During the first year of fellowship, the fellow is expected to

- Work 3 10-hour shifts per week in the emergency department under the direct supervision of faculty attending
- Do research and administrative work in the office for 2 days per week
- Attend weekly didactic presentations by the faculty on a combination of core curriculum and didactic topics for 2 hours

---

Box 2

Goals of The University of Texas MD Anderson Cancer Center Oncologic Emergency Fellowship

- Interpret the most common radiology, computed tomography, MRI, and PET findings encountered with patients with cancer who present to the emergency department.
- Manage complex hematological problems encountered with acutely ill oncology patients.
- Understand the treatment of neutropenic fever.
- Understand the current treatment modalities for most commonly treated cancers.
- Understand the common complications of radiation therapy and treatment of such complications.
- Perform ultrasound techniques used to diagnose common ailments of patients with cancer.
- Be proficient with thoracentesis, paracentesis, and airway management of patients with cancer.
- Participate in a scholarly activity project as defined by the program director.
- Participate in a quality improvement project.

- Attend faculty meetings that include a presentation of topical importance, as well as attend a certain proportion of graduate medical education (GME) core curriculum lecture series and GME competency lecture series on a weekly basis.

An optional second year is offered that includes a clinical track, as well as the opportunity to pursue a research project. The second year allows the fellow to enhance their clinical decision making in OEM, as well as obtain experience that will enhance the fellow's academic capabilities in a particular research area.

The OEM fellows practice under the direct supervision of faculty attending at all times and are aligned with mentors. The program director assesses trainee performance through biannual evaluations, faculty observation and feedback, and biannual program evaluation of the curriculum.

SUMMARY

The cancer population in the United States continues to grow and is projected to do so for the near future.[1,2] The current cancer population has a high rate of admission.[3] With this ever-increasing population and its unique disease processes, further training and knowledge may be needed in emergency departments in the future.

An ideal training program to accomplish this would strive to care for the patient as a whole. This may include treatment of the sequelae of the malignancy, progressive disease, symptom control, adverse effects, and the inclusion of palliative care. At this time, The Ohio State University and MD Anderson both have training programs in OEM. As the cancer population continues to grow, there may be further need for fellowship designs and implementation.

REFERENCES

1. Howlader N, Noone A, Krapcho M, et al. SEER cancer statistics review. 2017. Available at: https://seer.cancer.gov/csr/1975_2014/. Accessed October 27, 2017.
2. Bluethmann SM, Mariotto AB, Rowland JH. Anticipating the "silver tsunami": prevalence trajectories and comorbidity burden among older cancer survivors in the united states. Cancer Epidemiol Biomarkers Prev 2016;25(7):1029–36.

3. Rivera DR, Gallicchio L, Brown J, et al. Trends in adult cancer-related emergency department utilization: An analysis of data from the nationwide emergency department sample. JAMA Oncol 2017;3(10):e172450.
4. Wagner J, Arora S. Oncologic metabolic emergencies. Emerg Med Clin North Am 2014;32(3):509–25.
5. Khan UA, Shanholtz CB, McCurdy MT. Oncologic mechanical emergencies. Emerg Med Clin North Am 2014;32(3):495–508.
6. White L, Ybarra M. Neutropenic fever. Emerg Med Clin North Am 2014;32(3): 549–61.
7. Young JS, Simmons JW. Chemotherapeutic medications and their emergent complications. Emerg Med Clin North Am 2014;32(3):563–78.
8. Todd KH, Thomas CR Jr. An Inflection Point in the Evolution of Oncologic Emergency Medicine. Ann Emerg Med 2016;68:712–6.
9. Hill M, Okugo G. Emergency medicine physician attitudes toward HPV vaccine uptake in an emergency department setting. Hum Vaccin Immunother 2014;10: 2551–6.
10. Bernstein SL, Boudreaux ED, Cydulka RK, et al. Tobacco control interventions in the emergency department: a joint statement of emergency medicine organizations. Ann Emerg Med 2006;48:e417–26.
11. Hungerford DW, Pollock DA, Todd KH. Acceptability of emergency department–based screening and brief intervention for alcohol problems. Acad Emerg Med 2000;7:1383–92.
12. Hoffman JR, Mower WR, Wolfson AB, et al. Validation of a set of clinical criteria to rule out injury to the cervical spine in patients with blunt trauma. N Engl J Med 2000;343:94–9.
13. Mandelblatt J, Freeman H, Winczewski D, et al. Implementation of a breast and cervical cancer screening program in a public hospital emergency department. Cancer Control Center of Harlem. Ann Emerg Med 1996;28:493–8.
14. Trowbridge R, King R, Byun R, et al. Facilitating colon-rectal cancer screening among emergency department patients and visitors. Ann Emerg Med 2010;56: S104–5.
15. Fitch K, Pyenson B. Milliman client report. Cancer patients receiving chemotherapy: opportunities for better management. New York: Milliman Inc; 2010.
16. Advisory Board Company. Coordinating seamless transitions across care settings. Available at: https://www.advisory.com/research/oncology-roundtable/studies/2013/coordinating-seamless-transitions-across-care-settings. Accessed February 22, 2016.
17. Todd KH. Practically speaking: emergency medicine and the palliative care movement. Emerg Med Australas 2012;24:4–6.
18. Lamba S, Desandre PL, Todd KH, et al. Integration of palliative care into emergency department: the IPAL EM collaboration. J Emerg Med 2014;46:264–70.
19. EPEC. Emergency medicine: education in palliative and end-of-life care for emergency medicine. 2012. Available at: http://epec.net/epec_em.php?curid^1/45. Accessed February 22, 2016.
20. National Institutes of Health. NCI funding policy for RPG awards FY15. Available at: http://deainfo.nci.nih.gov/grantspolicies/FinalFundLtr.htm. Accessed February 22, 2016.

Moving?

Make sure your subscription moves with you!

To notify us of your new address, find your **Clinics Account Number** (located on your mailing label above your name), and contact customer service at:

Email: journalscustomerservice-usa@elsevier.com

800-654-2452 (subscribers in the U.S. & Canada)
314-447-8871 (subscribers outside of the U.S. & Canada)

Fax number: 314-447-8029

Elsevier Health Sciences Division
Subscription Customer Service
3251 Riverport Lane
Maryland Heights, MO 63043

*To ensure uninterrupted delivery of your subscription, please notify us at least 4 weeks in advance of move.

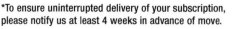
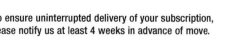

Printed and bound by CPI Group (UK) Ltd, Croydon, CR0 4YY

08/05/2025

01864727-0001